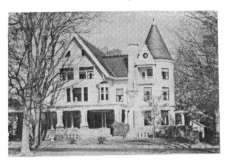

UNMASKING

UNMASKING
PMS

**The Complete PMS
Medical Treatment Plan**

JOSEPH MARTORANO, M.D.

and

MAUREEN MORGAN C.S.W., R.N.

with

WILLIAM FRYER

M. EVANS AND COMPANY, INC.
NEW YORK

The advice offered in this book, though based on the authors' considerable experience with thousands of patients, is not intended to be a substitute for the advice and counsel of your personal physician.

In order to better serve our patients and make the most appropriate clinical decisions, we have no financial interests in any of the substances we recommend including vitamins and progesterone.

Copyright © 1993 by Joseph Martorano M.D.; Maureen Morgan C.S.W., R.N.; and William Fryer

M. Evans and Company, Inc.
216 East 49th Street
New York, New York 10017

Library of Congress Cataloging-in-Publication Data

Martorano, Joseph T.
    Unmasking PMS : the complete PMS medical treatment plan / Joseph
Martorano, Maureen Morgan, and William Fryer.
      p. cm.
    Includes index.
    ISBN 0-87131-692-7 (cloth) : $21.95. — ISBN 0-87131-704-4 (pbk.) : $12.95
    1. Premenstrual syndrome—Popular works. I. Morgan, Maureen.
II. Fryer, William, 1949–   . III. Title.
RG165.M37   1993
618.1'72—dc20   93-72
                                                       CIP

Book design by Bernard Schleifer

Typesetting by AeroType, Inc.

Manufactured in the United State of America

9 8 7 6 5 4 3 2 1

We dedicate this book to the thousands of women whose stories deepened our knowledge of PMS and whose feedback refined our methods of healing them.

Contents

Acknowledgments   9

Introduction   13

PART I
Understanding PMS   17

    1. The Reality of PMS   19

    2. Tracking Down Your PMS   27

    3. Precipitating Factors and Differential Diagnosis   39

    4. Fueling Your Brain   51

Interlude: Six Helpful Hints for Better Sleep   61

PART II
Masks and Misdiagnosis   63

    5. PMS Depression   65

    6. Mood Swings and Manic Depression   81

    7. Anxiety and Tension   89

    8. Panic Attacks and Heart Problems   97

    9. Headaches   107

   10. Alcoholism   119

PART III
Other Conditions Related to the Hormonal Cycle   **127**

    11. Dysmenorrhea   129

    12. Postpartum Depression   135

    13. Menopause   141

Interlude: Fluid Retention   147

PART IV
The PMS Nutritional Treatment Plan   **151**

    14. Changing Your Life   153

    15. Nutritional Therapy for PMS   159

    16. Exercise Therapy for PMS   177

    17. Five Steps to Overcoming the Psychological
           Problems Associated with PMS   183

Interlude: PMS and Your Family   189

PART V
Beyond Nutrition Therapy   **191**

    18. Progesterone Therapy   193

    19. The Glucose Tolerance Test   201

    20. Drugs and Their Side Effects   207

    21. Treatment-Resistant PMS   217

    22. How to Find the Best Help for Your PMS   229

Index   235

Acknowledgments

There are far too many to adequately thank.

First of all, we'd like to recognize the ever growing, more cognizant women of America and an astute media health network that has enabled us to help so many thousands of women.

And we would like to acknowledge Dr. Norman Weiss, our co-founder, for his great support and welcome collaboration.

Then for their ever generous and sharing professionalism, we would like to thank our colleagues at PMS Access, specifically Treacy Colbert, Marla Ahlgrimm, and David Myers for their continuing assistance in developing a viable network for PMS patients in the United States, along with other colleagues like Stephanie Bender, Denise Sabal, and Niels Lauerson who have also blazed the path for treatment of PMS patients, and Dr. Turan Itil whose innovative brainmapping allowed us to demonstrate the effects of progesterone on the brain.

But this book could not have been written without Michael Cohn, our agent, whose stewardship provided welcome guidance, and George de Kay, a great editor, fine publisher, and good friend.

One of my patients, Sally S., once said to me, "You know what really upsets me?"

"This could all have been treated long ago. I could have been *happy* all these years."

Introduction

Over the years we've seen far too many women struggling through what ought to be the happiest and most productive period of their lives without a proper diagnosis of their problems. We've heard too many stories of bad treatment, broken marriages, ruined relationships, lost jobs, work curtailed or never undertaken, and of dreams stifled or put on hold because untreated PMS had undermined self-esteem and self-confidence.

We know there are millions of you out there who aren't getting the help you need and deserve. Instead you're often labeled "mentally ill" or "personality disordered" because PMS involves so many body systems that most physicians still don't recognize it. They see one or more of its many "masks" and treat these disguises instead of the real problem. If you dare to tell them their treatment didn't work, they too frequently see you as the problem.

For decades, in fact ever since the American medical establishment started collecting demographic data, statistics have revealed a consistently disproportionate number of women who sought treatment for migraines, anxiety disorders, panic attacks, and recurrent or treatment-resistant episodes of depression. We asked ourselves the following questions:

Why did women experience these problems so much more frequently than men? Was there something inherently more fragile about the female psyche? Did it in any way validate the Freudian hypothesis that women secretly "really longed" to be men and became depressed by their femininity, or does a woman's role in society set her up for anxiety and/or depression? Did women experience "raging hormones?" Did any of the above make them essentially unreliable?

Twelve years ago, we began our medical detective work, hoping to find the real answers and committed to assisting the women who came to us for help with these baffling problems.

The mainstream of the American medical establishment was for years dominated by a conservative, masculine-oriented chauvinism, that scarcely bothered to disguise its basic assumption that women were merely inferior versions of men, that they were more prone to break down psychologically, and that they were histrionic and unreliable reporters of their symptoms. In other words, women were not to be taken too seriously.

At first we scarcely had a clue as to how to argue convincingly against these assumptions. But as we collected our own data over the years, we began to see patterns. Women were actually reporting groupings of symptoms, and these groupings appeared to cluster at times. These occurrences spurred us on to try to find an explanation. Eventually we realized that the event about which the symptoms revolved was the menstrual cycle.

From this we came to be aware that the psychological disorders so disproportionately high in women were actually only symptoms of the underlying disorder, a phenomenon now known as Premenstrual Syndrome or PMS.

In the community of women in this country, few would say that PMS doesn't exist. But there are many women who suffer silently and publicly deny that they have PMS, for fear of lending credence to the myth that women are essentially unreliable because of their hormonal storms. Sadly for them, and for the truth, this position backfires. It is not women in general who evoke the stereotype of the "unreliable woman." It is the tiny—albeit highly visible—minority of women with the most severe untreated PMS who evoke and perpetuate that hated and inaccurate view of women.

And yet, more than twenty years after the syndrome was definitively defined by Katharina Dalton in London, the mainstream of American medicine continues to ignore—or dismiss as a "benign, self-limiting disorder"—this condition that disrupts the lives of women, their families, and their worlds in general.

Therefore, we felt we had to write this book to provide women with the real story: What PMS is; why it's so commonly missed, misdiagnosed, or mistreated by physicians; how PMS "masks" itself as many varied illnesses and disorders, and—most importantly—what you need to do to heal yourself from PMS.

Why are we uniquely qualified to take on this task?

We have been working in this area for more than twelve years. Dr. Martorano, a Board Certified psychiatrist specializing in psychopharmacology (drug treatment for psychiatric disorders), began noticing a pattern. Many women whom he evaluated before prescribing antidepressants for their depression (or tranquilizers for their tension and anxiety) did not really meet the criteria for the illness with which they had been diagnosed. Furthermore, these women did not respond as expected to the drugs prescribed for them. He began looking for other explanations and in doing so came across the work done by Dr. Katharina Dalton in London. After thoroughly researching her findings and after communicating with the two or three clinicians in the United States who were seeing women with these problems, he became convinced that PMS did exist and that its existence explained why women were diagnosed with depression, anxiety, and panic disorders so much more frequently than men.

Dalton and her American counterparts treated women diagnosed as having PMS with progesterone and vitamin therapy. Dr. Martorano began his search for a treatment plan that would rely on progesterone only for unresponsive PMS cases. He devised a holistic treatment protocol, and in June 1980, with Maureen Morgan and Dr. Norman Weiss as his co-founders, opened PMS Medical (at 141 East 55th Street, NY, NY 10022; telephone 212-751-3135), a private center for the diagnosis and treatment of PMS. We are still hard at work helping women.

In the following chapters we'll take you step-by-step through the areas of recognizing and stripping away the many masks of PMS. Then we'll instruct you in self-monitoring and self-diagnosis. In the third Part of the book we'll reveal our up-to-the-minute treatment formula that has helped thousands of women like you overcome their PMS and reclaim their self-esteem, their work, and their lives. We'll help you to learn how to become expert at helping yourself. We'll help you to recognize when, and if, you may need a medical expert to assist in your treatment; and we'll help you to learn how to choose a physician and how to become a competent, self-confident, informed consumer of medical services. We'll help you to handle the social and work ramifications of PMS and give you guidance to help you share your concerns and needs with family members, so that they can understand and support you.

We've got the help you need, but our knowledge alone won't do the trick. Just as when you become competent at any other complicated skill, the experts can give you useful advice, but you've got to do the actual work. You've got to make the necessary changes. We know you can do it. We've seen so many other women heal themselves from PMS. Through this book, we'll be right there beside you as you take each step.

Let's get started now, you've already suffered too long!

UNDERSTANDING PMS

1

The Reality of PMS

PMS is prevalent. PMS is epidemic. PMS involves tens of millions of women. PMS disrupts the lives of a significant percentage of the female population who has it, and adversely affects the lives of the men, women, and children who love them, live with them, and work with them. But there's no doubt that although very common among women from fifteen to fifty-five, PMS is the most frequently misdiagnosed and mistreated illness in America today.

Why do so many well-educated, well-intentioned physicians miss or misdiagnose PMS? To begin with, women's complaints are frequently dismissed. There is a misperception, still present in our medical community, that women are preoccupied with their health. Women are not taken as seriously as men, and consequently doctors frequently don't listen carefully enough when their patients are female.

Furthermore, PMS is often masked by misleading symptoms; it can appear in any combination of more than 140 different signs and symptoms. PMS can involve so many symptoms in the body that many physicians, trained as specialists, refer their PMS patients to another doctor because they don't feel equipped to deal with the many symptoms outside their area.

Getting Past Freud

Finally, in many cases the physician decides that anyone with so many symptoms must need psychiatric help. Nowadays, whenever a woman has an elusive, hard-to-diagnose symptom, physicians generally deem that it must be psychological. Once a woman speaks of anxiety, tension, or depression, she is shuttled into the mental health system, where her physiological complaints are largely ignored.

The thrust of this book will be three-pronged. We will teach you to recognize and strip away the many myths and masks of PMS. Then we'll equip you to diagnose your own disorder. Finally, we'll give you a comprehensive treatment program that has brought relief to thousands of women like you who have been treated at our PMS Center.

Searching for Help

Typically, the PMS Center patient comes to us after seeing five previous doctors and spending close to five thousand dollars on ineffective care. Mistreatment ranges from the subtle to the devastating, from the seemingly reasonable to the patently absurd.

Most of the time, the *masks* of PMS are the problem. PMS normally travels in disguise. Its disguises are numerous and doctors are often fooled by its disguises. A woman with a straightforward, thoroughly treatable case of PMS is often diagnosed as depressive or anxious. You might reasonably assume that such a misdiagnosis is no more than a temporary, minor difficulty. Unfortunately, that's not usually the case. Simply put, *the vast majority of American physicians are ill-informed and ill-educated when it comes to PMS.* And what they *don't* know can certainly hurt you.

The Superficial Diagnosis

For instance, you go to a doctor and get a superficial surface diagnosis . . . not exactly an incorrect diagnosis but one that doesn't establish the etiology, or cause, of the disorder. You tell the doctor you feel "anxious." He or she agrees that you appear especially anxious. But does he or she look for the cause of your anxiety? What if it is caused by PMS or even a sensitivity to a nasal spray such as phenylpropylalanine, which causes anxiety in many women? *What is the correct diagnosis?*

Or maybe something really steers you wrong, like the chest pains you experience when you have panic attacks. Your heart beats so fast that you think it is going to fly out of your chest. And you go to the doctor. He examines you and does a cardiogram, which is negative, though your heart rate accelerates at times. Then he does a sonogram, which is also negative, but he believes you have a slight heart murmur. "Quite mild," he insists. "It may be indicative of mitral valve prolapse." In that moment, your whole world darkens. You've heard the magical word "heart" and you go into a state of intensified anxiety.

You limit your activities, stop your exercise, and surprisingly, the panic attacks increase. *But is mitral valve prolapse the correct diagnosis?* You may actually have a masked case of PMS, and, if you do, the misinformation and the "help" you've received will only make your anxiety worse.

You can unmask PMS if you know exactly what questions from Chapter 22 to ask your doctor.

That's the reason for writing this book: using our extensive clinical experience developed from years of *listening* to case histories like yours, we can offer you a complete system that will allow you to avoid misdiagnosis and mistreatment.

The Range of Misdiagnosis

Our patients have been misdiagnosed in every way that women can be misdiagnosed—and often with the aid of complex and expensive tests. After the specialists had worked them up, many of these future patients of ours were worried about brain tumors, or multiple sclerosis, or insanity. Neurologists searched their brains with CAT scans and MRIs, while gynecologists searched their reproductive organs. Most frequently, however, they were treated by psychologists, psychiatrists, or therapists for their "disturbed" mental state. Much of PMS—tension, depression, irritability, and unpredictable, meteoric mood swings—appears psychological, especially if the mental health professional is unaware of the masks of PMS.

In spite of that appearance, and so many other false appearances, the truth is that the Premenstrual Syndrome is a hormonal disorder and has to do with the imbalance of estrogen and progesterone, the two major female hormones, during the weeks before your period. Neither your nerves nor your genitals—not even your thoughts—are significantly involved in treating the problem. PMS and hormones are inextricably linked.

The balance of hormones in the body is a delicate one. Nonetheless the majority of women (60 percent) are sufficiently well tuned that they don't feel the sort of discomfort that would cause them to seek help. They go from menarche to menopause without incident. To these women, PMS is not a reality. But 40 percent of all women in the childbearing years *do* have significant problems, and 10 to 12 percent of women experience such intense PMS that it disrupts their lives and the lives of family, friends, and co-workers.

If you're a woman with such severe PMS, then each month during your premenstruum, you're acutely miserable, difficult to live with, and tormented by a wide variety of physical and psychological symptoms that are too much for any one person to cope with.

It's important for you to get the help you need. If you aren't treated effectively for a condition as serious as PMS, your quality of life can suffer catastrophic consequences.

Why Is PMS So Hard to Diagnose?

There is compelling evidence that most PMS sufferers are not yet getting effective treatment. *Is it because no one understands how to care for PMS, because the disorder is mysterious?* Once upon a time that was true, but now it's absolutely not the case. Proper diagnosis can be made without costly tests, and good care can and should be standard.

American doctors are largely at fault, even if the fault lies largely in their education. Effective methods of handling PMS were developed in Great Britain more than thirty years ago. Why aren't American doctors treating their PMS patients according to the tried-and-true methods developed in England during the 1960s and 1970s? Why are we so backward and behind the times?

We've noticed that doctors who don't treat their PMS patients correctly generally fall into three groups:

The uninformed. By this time, just about every physician in the country knows about PMS, but a majority still have very little idea of how to treat it. Their ability to diagnose the disorder is primitive at best. Their knowledge of diet is superficial. And, if they've heard about natural progesterone for PMS, they have a marked tendency to confuse it with the synthetic form, which not only doesn't work but in the long run can actually worsen the symptoms it's supposed to be improving.

The dismissive. This less than benevolent group simply shrugs off the pain of their patients. They're most often physicians with a grin-and-bear-it mentality. They usually perceive female patients as "complainers." To these misogynists PMS is due to the inherent defective character of the woman rather than to her hormonal imbalance.

The opportunistic. These are the doctors who treat patients only with the treatment practiced in their own specialty and apparently are not concerned by the dismal ineffectiveness of this treatment when it's applied to PMS. Shamefully, although most doctors want their patients to get well, sometimes the doctor's needs overshadow the patient's. These needs include keeping their self-esteem intact, keeping a practice going, making money, and feeling comfortable with the sort of medicine they're practicing— and that usually requires that any particular disorder they treat be put within their frame of reference.

Unfortunately, no matter how and why the doctor misses PMS, this translates into bad medicine. PMS is an illness that manifests itself through hundreds of different symptoms, as you'll see in the next chapter. First let's take a brief look at the history of PMS and its treatment.

A Short History of PMS

It took a very long time for PMS to be "discovered." Presumably, as far back as the cave dwellers, some women found themselves growing irritable and depressed during the weeks before menstruation. Presumably, their feet swelled and their breasts were tender and their tolerance for the foibles and follies of their mates grew very slim. However, before the twentieth century, no one had any idea that there was such a thing as PMS.

The disorder was finally described more than sixty years ago by Dr. Robert T. Frank. In 1931, he produced a paper entitled "The Hormonal Causes of Premenstrual Tension," which correctly outlined the physiological and psychological changes that he had observed in women during the premenstrual portion of their cycle. He also surmised that changes in the progesterone level were very likely to be responsible for much of what he was seeing.

In 1925, six years before Frank's important discovery, Drs. R. Okey and E. L. Robb reported that glucose tolerance curves were abnormal for women during menstruation and that women sometimes showed tendencies toward *low blood sugar*. In 1944, Dr. Seale Harris, one of the pioneers in the study of hypoglycemia, reported in the *Southern Medical Journal* that women frequently experience hunger, fatigue, nervousness, and sweating immediately prior to menstruation. These were solid findings made by competent physicians but the medical establishment failed to see their importance and never took them seriously.

The next four decades continued to be grim for women with PMS. In their search for relief, they were given useless treatments, were told they needed a vacation, needed a job, needed more children, needed more sex, needed more time away from their children, needed a glass or two of wine to help them relax, or needed a tranquilizer to soothe their feminine psyche. And, increasingly often, they were told they needed a psychiatrist.

Meanwhile, in England, Katharina Dalton, who earned her medical degree in 1948, was about to become the mother of modern PMS treatment and diagnosis. Dr. Dalton's own premenstrual experiences led her to speculate on the effects this portion of the female cycle had upon women.

The splitting migraine headaches she got each month before her period made her reexamine the complaints of many of her patients. Dalton wrote the first paper in British medical literature on PMS, in collaboration with Dr. Raymond Greene, in 1953. By that time, it was already clear to her that PMS was a medical disorder that is hormonally related.

Dr. Dalton was nothing if not persistent. She soon established a clinic in London to treat the condition, and, by the late 1960s, PMS was no longer a strange or an exotic illness in the minds of the British medical community. In England, PMS was accepted not as a psychiatric problem but as a hormonal disorder.

Dalton came to the United States in August 1979 to help publicize the condition, and controversy flared. Over the next several years, medical articles and media attention made PMS a household word. The first American center for treating PMS opened in Boston and a remarkable national network of women began to campaign for the medical acceptance of PMS.

An astonished and markedly unenthusiastic American medical establishment watched uncertainly as PMS broke like a wave over its hitherto indifferent shoulders. Hormone disorder? Depression, mood swings, migraines bringing about endocrine changes in the premenstrual portion of the month? Surely all that was exaggerated, if it was even real. And sadly, some misguided feminists, in the interest of preserving the myth that men and women are not merely equal but the *same*, persist in declaring that PMS just doesn't exist.

Indeed PMS has often been handled as if it were a political "hot potato" rather than a legitimate medical disorder. Many women have concluded that to acknowledge the existence of a disorder that impairs the judgement of even a small number of women would lend credence to the claims of hostile males anxious to suggest that women are unreliable because of their inherent "raging hormones." Ironically, it may well be that severe, untreated cases of PMS provided the stereotype in the first place.

The interesting thing about PMS is that scientifically speaking, there ought to be very little that is controversial about it.

- PMS can be directly observed in the behavior of millions of women during the days preceding their period.
- PMS can usually be treated with a better than 90 percent rate of success.
- PMS is not in your imagination, but it can be shown that it *is* in your brain. We can say this now because the effects of PMS and the rapid results of treating it can be observed through a dramatic new technique called *brain mapping*.

PMS is now on the medical map. Only the most hidebound and unprogressive doctors still deny its existence. Perhaps the next thing is to try to help them to understand what causes it. So let's look at the next chapter. Even if you can't convince your physician to read that chapter, you'll find that it has an immensely clarifying effect on your sense of your own body. Remember, *you* may be the most important PMS doctor you're ever going to have.

2

Tracking Down Your PMS

THIS CHAPTER WILL SHOW YOU:

- The many and varied symptoms of PMS
- One woman's ordeal of misdiagnosis
- How to keep your menstrual calendar
- How to determine if you have PMS

As we have said, PMS manifests itself through hundreds of different symptoms. Look at this following list:

Common PMS Symptoms

Which Ones Do You Have?

    Abdominal bloating or swelling
    Acne
    Angry outbursts
    Anxiety
    Appetite changes
    Asthmatic attacks
    Avoidance of social activities
    Backache
    Bladder irritation
    Bleeding gums
    Breast swelling/tenderness

Bruising
Clumsiness
Confusion
Conjunctivitis
Constipation
Cramps, pelvic
Craving salty foods
Craving sweet foods
Crying spells
Decreased hearing
Decreased productivity at school or work
Decreased sex drive
Depression
Distractibility
Dizziness
Drowsiness
Dull abdominal pain
Eye pain
Facial swelling
Fatigue
Fear of going out alone (agoraphobia)
Fear of losing control
Finger swelling
Food sensitivity
Forgetfulness
Generalized aches and pains
Headaches
Herpes (cold sores)
Hives or rashes
Hot flashes
Increased alcohol consumption/sensitivity
Increased sensitivity to light
Increased sensitivity to noise
Inefficiency
Indecision
Insomnia
Irritability
Joint pains

Leg cramps
Leg swelling
Mood swings
Mouth sores
Muscle aches or tenderness
Nausea
Palpitations
Panic attacks
Poor coordination
Poor judgment
Poor memory
Poor vision
Restlessness
Ringing in ears
Runny nose
Seizures
Sinusitis
Sore throat
Spots in front of eyes
Suspiciousness
Tearfulness
Tension
Tingling in hands and feet
Tremors
Visual changes
Vomiting
Weight gain

That's a lot of possibly complex symptoms, and that's one of the reasons why doctors frequently have difficulty in diagnosing PMS. Here are three other reasons:

1. *There is no definitive diagnostic test that confirms a diagnosis of PMS.* Many doctors are too dependent on highly specific laboratory tests to confirm the presence of disease and are reluctant to depend on a really thorough history.

2. *PMS has no specific age of onset.* Women have it anywhere from menarche to menopause. It usually has a gradual insidious onset making it more difficult to diagnose.
3. *There is no clear course of development.* The number of days and symptoms and the type of severity of symptoms can vary greatly from month to month, even in the same patient.

Given all these variables, how can anyone possibly diagnose PMS? The answer is in its timing. *The crucial fact about PMS is that symptoms appear only in the premenstrual portion of the month—or, if they appear throughout the month, are consistently worse in the premenstrual period. The symptoms will decrease or subside completely at—or slightly after—menstruation occurs each month.*

The Case of Sarah R.

Let's look at the misdiagnosis and mistreatment of one woman. Sarah R., age thirty-four, is married and has two children. Her PMS has been getting worse for some time now. Her breasts ache, her body swells in the premenstruum, she's irritable and often angry at that time of the month. She also gets depressed at times.

Sarah's family doctor hasn't been much help, so she makes an appointment with her gynecologist. Dr. Y. is a very busy doctor with a well-deserved reputation. During her two pregnancies, Sarah always found him diligent, fair, and competent. She goes to see him on a Tuesday for an extensive consultation.

Sarah is embarrassed, almost ashamed, to tell him how badly incapacitated she is each month, and how demoralizing, for herself and everyone around her, her angry outbursts can be. She only hints at her secret—the fact that for two or three days each month, she is so paralyzed by depression that she can't function even up to her most minimally acceptable standards. Nonetheless, he gets the basic picture.

Dr. Y. gives her a thorough gynecological exam, always a good idea to "rule out" any other disease possibilities. When he's done, he says, "Good news, your exam is negative."

Sarah looks at him blankly. Since she wants a solution, this doesn't really sound like good news. "So what do I do now?" she finally asks.

He informs her that it's important to have a good diet with lots of vitamin B_6.

"What's a good diet?"

"Avoid alcohol and sugar," he tells her—which is excellent advice as far as it goes.

"Is wine O.K.?"

"In limited amounts," he answers. That's a bad answer, one that Dr. Y. would never give if he really understood PMS.

She asks him about her swollen breasts and the awful fluid retention she suffers monthly.

His answer is a diuretic to reduce fluid in the body. And now Dr. Y reaches for his prescription pad, an action that almost always makes a doctor feel better. "Hydrodiuril®, 25 mgs. a day," he writes.

Well, Sarah tries it, and it does reduce swelling, but it also results in adding overwhelming fatigue to her list of complaints because of the potassium that's being lost from her body along with excess fluid.

Dr. Y. gives her potassium supplements. Her other PMS symptoms have also improved a little bit because she has cut out sugar as he suggested. But then, on the night of her tenth anniversary, she goes to a neighborhood restaurant with her husband, and they order a bottle of fine champagne to celebrate. Within two hours all of the worst emotional consequences of PMS are alive and on the loose. Shouting and misery.

She calls Dr. Y. for an emergency appointment the following morning, and when she gets to see him mentions that she's heard about progesterone.

"So have I," the doctor says and reaches for the ever present prescription pad. "Provera®, 10 mgs. twice a day," he writes.

She tries it, and briefly gets better. Unfortunately, in prescribing Provera®, Dr. Y. has mistaken synthetic progesterone for natural progesterone. While the synthetic form brings some initial relief, it actually starts Sarah on a downward spiral by blocking natural progesterone from acting on the appropriate receptor sites in her brain.

Sarah gets worse, and she and her husband have more angry disagreements. Her depression deepens to such an extent that a day or two before her period, she sometimes has fleeting but frightening suicidal thoughts. Her self-esteem is all but gone. She feels like she's losing herself.

Sarah calls Dr. Y. again. He is thoroughly puzzled. It is obviously time for her to move on to the endocrinologists, the internists, the lay therapists, and the psychiatrists. And, in the years before we saw her, that was exactly what Sarah did.

How to Avoid Misdiagnosis

By now you are probably saying: Could something like that happen in the enlightened 1990s? How likely is it to happen to me? The answer is that it is happening all the time. Sad to say, you are far more likely to repeat Sarah's experience than be immediately offered appropriate care for your PMS.

Misdiagnosis is the crucial factor in the mistreatment of Premenstrual Syndrome. Misdiagnosis followed by mistreatment is the common fate. None of this has to be your fate!

Keeping a Menstrual Calendar

PMS is eminently treatable. If your doctor hasn't been able to help you, there is a great deal you can do to help yourself.

Your first step will be to get a calendar. Most of the time a calendar is a better diagnostic tool for PMS than thousands of dollars worth of lab tests.

By using a menstrual calendar to *accurately* record symptoms over a long enough period to provide a fair sample (usually three months), you can readily see *which symptoms cluster in the premenstrual part of the cycle*. Though a seemingly simple device, the menstrual calendar can yield an incredible amount of helpful data.

From it you'll not only learn if some of your symptoms are caused by PMS, but also which problems are not PMS-induced. You'll even find problems that exist throughout the entire month but get worse during the premenstrual portion.

HOW TO USE YOUR CALENDAR
TO FRAME YOUR SYMPTOMS

Fill in your calendar each day. Relying on memory leads to mistakes. Record three separate sets of information on your calendar.

1. *Make a daily record of your symptoms.* Record any symptoms of ill health, emotional changes, or pain that you experience, using a designated letter for each symptom (for example, H for headache, B for bloat, etc.) Then make a record of your overall mood each day, rating it on a scale of 0 to 10, with 0 representing extreme depression and 10 feeling fine.
2. *Keep a record of which days you menstruate (flow).* Mark the days of full menstruation with a large M. If the flow is very slight, use a small m. You will probably find some variation in your menstrual cycle. Not everyone has a twenty-eight day cycle. That is just the average. Normal cycles can range from as short as twenty-one days to as long as thirty-six days.
3. *It's very important to know that your other symptoms may not be so clear-cut.* Record them anyway with an appropriate notation like a "?". And when you are quite clear about whether a particular physical or mental state is present, use a 0 to 3 scale to measure severity, with 3 representing a

MONTHLY MENSTRUAL CALENDAR

1   2   3

DAY	SYMPTOMS MOOD	WT	SYMPTOMS MOOD	WT	SYMPTOMS MOOD	WT
1						
2						
3						
4						
5						
6						
7						
8						
9						
10						
11						
12						
13						
14						
15						
16						
17						
18						
19						
20						
21						
22						
23						
24						
25						
26						
27						
28						
29						
30						
31						

symptom-free state: 2 = mild, 1 = moderate, 0 = severe. These measurements of intensity are important because they make it possible for you to make a quantified comparison of your condition at different times of the menstrual month.

Your calendar will make it perfectly clear to you why the following definition fits:

PMS is a hormonal disorder characterized by the monthly recurrence of certain physical or psychological symptoms during the two weeks before menstruation, and the subsiding of these symptoms when flow begins or slightly afterwards.

Stripping the Masks of PMS

You've already learned that PMS is a disorder characterized by an incredibly varied number of symptoms. You realize that it can be identified most clearly by the timing of symptoms. And you're aware of the great probability that most physicians you go to for help will misdiagnose you unless you help them.

The masking misdiagnosises of PMS are too varied to note, but here's a list of the most common ones:

- anxiety and tension
- depression
- migraine headaches
- seizures
- alcoholism
- panic attacks
- agoraphobia (sometimes more mildly diagnosed as mood swings)
- eating disorders
- various personality disorders

Since PMS can mimic any or all of these, have sympathy for your doctor, even while you keep a firm hold on your calendar—it can be your lifeline to sanity.

We'd like you to look with us at some of the symptoms that may signify that PMS is a part of your life.

We've developed fifteen "marker" questions that can give you some idea of how likely it is that you have PMS.

1. Have three or more of the symptoms listed on pages 27–29 occurred during the week before your period for at least the past three months?
2. Do you gain weight or need a larger bra or dress size premenstrually?
3. Do you have seven or more consecutive days free of these symptoms each month after your period?
4. Did you experience side effects (depression, irritability, etc.) or worsening of your symptoms during or following the use of oral contraceptives?
5. Did the onset of your symptoms occur or increase after one of the following events: missed periods, hysterectomy, pregnancy, miscarriage, abortion, tubal ligation, major stress in your life?
6. Did your symptoms get worse after any of the above events?
7. Do you gain more than three pounds each month before your period?
8. Do your eating habits change noticeably during the time of your symptoms? Do you crave sugar, sweets, chocolate, etc.? Do you crave salt or salty foods?
9. Do you drink more during your symptom period or are you more sensitive to alcohol premenstrually?
10. If you've been pregnant, did you experience depression following the birth of your children?
11. Do you have to alter your life because of your premenstrual symptoms?
12. Is your productivity or quality of work impaired premenstrually?
13. Have you altered your career plans because you fear your symptoms may cause you to be unsuccessful?
14. Do you experience problems with friends or family members because of your symptoms?

The Words That Go With the Symptoms

These are some typical statements we've heard over and over from women with PMS.

"I want to be alone, and sometimes I cry for no reason at all."

"I get so irritable that no one can say anything to me."

"I get so tired that I think I can't go on, and I go on food binges that make me crazy."

"I'm frightened or anxious over little things, and my heart begins to pound."

"My body swells up so much I can hardly put my shoes on."

"I become so terribly depressed that sometimes I wonder if life is worth living."

"I panic when the kids get little bumps or bruises."

"I magnify every little problem."

"Each month when my period comes and my doubts and fears go away, I breathe a sigh of relief and hope it's over . . . and then, like clockwork, it starts again . . . I feel like I'm losing my mind."

15. Do you tend to forget or minimize the extent of the problems your symptoms caused, only to find that they return or even become worse the next month?

If you answered "yes" to more than five of these questions, you *probably* have PMS.

Where Do We Go From Here?

There are a number of aspects of PMS that we'd like to tell you about in this opening section of the book. The next chapter describes the major female life changes that can often precipitate PMS. Then the chapter after that covers low blood sugar, or hypoglycemia, and how it relates to mood and other symptoms. It's a subject you'll need to know about because, more than any other factor, this metabolic state is responsible for the most common premenstrual symptoms.

Once you've finished this part of the book you'll be well prepared to move on to Part II for a more detailed look at the misdiagnosis, or, as we call them, the masks of Premenstrual Syndrome. Often through stories of real people, you'll learn about symptoms that you may never have connected to your menstrual cycle but which may prove on examination—with a little calendar work—to be closely tied in to your PMS. In Part III we'll move on to other conditions related to the hormonal cycle including postpartum depression, dysmenorrhea, and menopause. Then in Part IV, we'll give you our complete PMS treatment plan. Finally, Part V will provide you with an overview of progesterone therapy and information on how to handle treatment-resistant PMS.

We think you'll find that the discoveries you're going to be making are fascinating. We hope that they've already begun to change how you see your PMS and yourself.

3

Precipitating Factors and Differential Diagnosis

THIS CHAPTER WILL SHOW YOU:

- How your hormones work as part of the female reproductive cycle
- Six common hormonal events that can precipitate the hormonal imbalance that leads to PMS
- How to start diagnosing PMS, so that you can distinguish between it and other conditions
- The most frequent confusing disorders

We're going to take a detailed look at the factors that can precipitate Premenstrual Syndrome. PMS begins at different times in different women's lives, and often there's a very specific reason for its onset. Clearly, it's useful for you to know these reasons. You'll find that most of them are related to the delicate balance of your hormonal cycle.

In the second half of this chapter we'll show you how you can distinguish between health disorders caused by PMS and those resulting from some other health problem in your life. In medicine, such a vital distinction is called making a *differential diagnosis*. Just as a person with a headache wants to be sure that his pain isn't caused by a brain tumor or an aneurysm, so you'll want to feel confident that you've distinguished between PMS and any other diagnosis. Until you've gained a certain amount of knowledge about PMS, that can be quite difficult to do. But once you know more it will be easier, and it really will make a tremendous difference in your life.

Hormones and You

Hormonal interactions during the menstrual cycle are delicate and complicated. Let's review the normal release of hormones during an average menstrual cycle as a prelude to understanding what can go wrong and how and when this can happen.

THE MENSTRUAL PHASE (DAYS 1–5)

As the menstrual flow from the previous cycle occurs, the next cycle begins. Estrogen and progesterone are at low levels, signaling the brain (the hypothalmus and pituitary) to begin secreting their stimulating hormones Luteinizing Hormone (LH) and Follicle Stimulating Hormone (FSH). This prompts the ovaries to begin a new reproductive cycle. FSH stimulates the development of a follicle, which will eventually become a ripened egg, within the ovary. LH stimulates the ovaries to produce estrogen.

THE PROLIFERATIVE/FOLLICULAR PHASE (DAYS 6–12)

LH and estrogen levels continue to rise, signaling the pituitary to cut back FSH production. Rising estrogen primes the pituitary to secrete LH.

THE PROLIFERATIVE PHASE (DAYS 12–13)

Estrogen production surges, leading to an increase in LH. Then estrogen falls off and FSH increases.

OVULATION (DAY 14)

Within 36 hours of the LH surge, the ovarian follicle releases its ripe egg and ovulation occurs. The site of the ruptured follicle undergoes a process called luteinization and becomes the corpus luteum, the place where the hormone progesterone is produced. This hormone prepares the lining of the uterus to support a fertilized egg, should one appear.

THE LUTEAL PHASE (DAYS 15–27)

This is the second half of the cycle. Progesterone continues to rise while FSH drops to its lowest level in the cycle. There is also a sharp decrease in LH. Progesterone peaks at about Day 22 if the egg is not fertilized. The corpus luteum shrinks and the progesterone level drops off. The lining of the uterus begins to break down and loosen. By Day 27 estrogen, progesterone, FSH, and LH are all at their lowest levels.

MENSTRUATION BEGINS (DAY 28)

The beginning of the flow becomes the next cycle's Day 1.

You can surely see how any disruption of hormonal interaction can lead to problems in the timing of the appearance or in the amount of the hormone present. Since each sequential hormone is triggered by the level of its predecessor, any failure or defect in the system can set the stage for the development of PMS.

Paths to PMS

Now you understand just how crucial it is that the balance of estrogen and progesterone in your body remain correct. A very large percentage of the women who have PMS didn't develop the disorder until something in their lives interfered with the pituitary-ovarian feedback loop, and drove their natural supply of progesterone down.

There are a number of common precipitating factors:

1. *Oral contraceptives.* The use of oral contraceptives is among the top five precipitants of Premenstrual Syndrome. At one time it was believed that birth control pills were an effective treatment for PMS, but now we know better. It's very likely that the initial confusion came about because doctors and their patients were mixing up the unpleasant symptoms of PMS with the unpleasant experience of menstrual cramps or dysmenorrhea. Oral contraceptives, composed of large amounts of estrogen, often do help to relieve menstrual cramps. This benefit is offset by many severe side effects not the least of which is a worsening of existing PMS symptoms or the precipitation of PMS.

If you are under thirty and the use of an oral contraceptive was associated with such unpleasant premenstrual side effects as headache, depression, bloating, and weight gain, then consider stopping the oral contraceptive and waiting a minimum of two months to evaluate your PMS. *Note: Be sure that you use an alternate method of contraception.*

Many doctors still believe that oral contraceptives are useful in the management of PMS. There is a good reason for this unfortunate confusion. Quite apart from their being behind the times, they have probably heard that progesterone may help PMS, and they know that contraceptives contain synthetic progesterone. When they prescribe the Pill for your PMS, they are prescribing that synthetic form. The results can be disastrous.

Synthetic progesterone, though it sometimes produces an initial good response, is not what your body needs. Even worse, it competes for the same receptor sites in your brain that natural progesterone uses. Thus, your brain may not even get to use the already inadequate supplies of progesterone that your body is producing during your premenstruum. Your PMS not only doesn't get better, it usually begins to get worse if you're on synthetic progesterone (progestogens).

If you have PMS, avoid oral contraceptives and all other forms of synthetic progesterone (if at all possible).

2. *Pregnancies.* Although we are hardly going to advise you to avoid having children, the fact is that pregnancy—especially multiple pregnancies—is one of the most potent precipitating events for Premenstrual Syndrome. Many women feel wonderful during their pregnancies, and the body's extremely high levels of progesterone is one of the reasons for this. But, not surprisingly, such a hormonally intense experience as pregnancy produces some permanent changes in the balance of hormones in the body. When those hormonal changes cause PMS, there is often an early warning sign shortly after the birth of the baby: *postpartum depression*. Approximately 7 to 10 percent of new mothers have very severe cases of postpartum depression. Women who have such depressions are often already PMS sufferers. However, Dr. Katharina Dalton has concluded from her studies that a woman who has not yet suffered PMS has a 90 percent chance of developing it after she experiences postpartum depression.

3. *Miscarriages and abortions.* These cause a sudden decrease in progesterone levels just as childbirth does. (Frequent miscarriages are often due to a relative lack of progesterone.)

4. *Tubal ligations.* This is a greatly overlooked precipitator of PMS. Some studies show that as many as 37 percent of women who have tubal ligations develop PMS and other complications, such as pelvic pain and irregular menstrual bleeding, following their surgery. Studies have shown that after tubal ligation women have higher estrogen and lower progesterone levels in the second half of their menstrual cycles—and that is the formula for PMS.

5. *Hysterectomies.* As you're probably aware, a shocking number of unnecessary hysterectomies are performed each year. In fact, the removal of the uterus is the most commonly performed major surgery for women in the United States. At least a third of these uteruses are essentially healthy. Women have their uteruses removed not merely to treat cancer—which is, of course, a very sound indication of the need for a hysterectomy—but to deal with uncontrollable dysmenorrhea (menstrual pain), myomas (tumors

CLINICAL CLUES

Answering the following questions can help you with your differential diagnosis.

- Was your PMS made worse by pregnancy? Did it get worse with subsequent pregnancies?
- Have you had repeated miscarriages during the first three months of pregnancy?
- Did your symptoms start after postpartum depression?
- Did you feel better during the second and third trimesters (the last six months) of your pregnancy?
- Did you have a bad reaction to oral contraceptives? Did you experience headache, weight gain, or depression?
- Do some of your symptoms occur when you have a long gap between meals?
- Do your symptoms wake you up in the middle of the night? And do you find that this is especially the case when you've gone a very long time without eating?
- Are you a Jekyll and Hyde? That is, *do you feel like an entirely different person once you ovulate, and again once you start menstruating?*

These are all signs of PMS!

consisting largely of muscle tissue), fibromas (benign tumors consisting of fibrous tissue), and repeated episodes of breakthrough bleeding (which can cause anemia). Sometimes women have hysterectomies to cure their Premenstrual Syndrome. This is particularly ill-advised, since it doesn't work.

Even worse, a hysterectomy may increase PMS or may precipitate it in a woman who has never had it before. Removing the uterus does not end the functioning of a woman's hormonal system. Hormones are still produced, but now they function erratically. A sudden and severe eruption of PMS symptoms following a hysterectomy is not uncommon. A woman who never had PMS may find she now has mood swings, depression, backache, and other PMS problems. She may find that her hormones are still released by the pituitary and the ovaries according to a monthly menstrual cycle even though she no longer menstruates.

PMS is not an indication for having a hysterectomy!

Do not be responsible for mistreating yourself by choosing to have hysterectomies, tubal ligations, and other progesterone-disturbing procedures unless you have very sound medical/personal reasons and you have carefully considered the possible consequences.

6. *Age.* Though some women have PMS symptoms in their teens, in general PMS is more common as women grow older and becomes most prevalent when they reach their thirties. Age changes the body, and the general pattern of hormonal change is toward the production of *less* progesterone. Since estrogen levels do not go down, an estrogen-progesterone imbalance is likely and so is PMS.

Have You Diagnosed PMS Correctly?

Of course, if you've read this far in the book, you probably believe you have Premenstrual Syndrome. If your symptoms occur only in the premenstrual portion of your cycle, it is very likely you're correct.

Ninety percent of the women who come to us for treatment of their PMS have self-diagnosed it. This is unfortunate because it means that most of the time their doctors *weren't diagnosing their problem*. The doctors were looking at some one symptom of their PMS and making the *wrong* differential diagnosis. A symptom or a series of symptoms were masking PMS. The histories that women give can be quite complex.

Take the case of Clare L., a thirty-five year old bookkeeper. Clare had been treated with diuretics for years, resulting in a persistent tiredness and profound weakness. Eventually she sought psychiatric help for her unexplained fatigue. Her original problem, premenstrual fluid retention, had now taken on a new mask through inappropriate treatment. In fact, the original problem had been virtually forgotten. Now the treatment was for her fatigue. Her psychiatrist concluded that she had an underlying depression, some unresolved problem in her intrapsychic life. He tried psychotherapy but after some months had to admit he was not effectively treating her "depression" this way. He turned to a common antidepressant, Elavil®. This had results!

Her fatigue got worse, she became sleepy, constipated, and dizzy. He had warned her about side effects, and antidepressants take some time to have their desired effect. Poor Clare was going to have to endure for a while. (See chapter 5 for more information on antidepressants and the misdiagnosis of depression.)

Eventually, there were more medications, more side effects, more diagnoses. Medicine can get pretty complicated when you make the wrong diagnosis to begin with. Layer after layer of misdiagnosis and mistreatment obscures the truth. It's almost like putting on makeup—eventually the original symptoms are almost totally hidden by the treatment.

Clare finally got the proper treatment, but we've heard hundreds of horror stories like hers. We can tell you some good news. In the past five years we've seen a dramatic increase in accurate referrals from psychotherapists who are becoming aware of the possibility of PMS when they're making their diagnoses. This gives us hope, for as we so often emphasize, misdiagnosis is the bane of the PMS sufferer.

Making a Differential Diagnosis

As important as establishing *what PMS is* is establishing *what PMS is not*. Work closely with your menstrual calendar and see if you have any symptoms that appear throughout the month and show no significant increase in the premenstruum. Don't be surprised if there are symptoms that exist throughout the month that get worse before your period. Some chronic diseases and disorders undergo intensification in relation to the menstrual cycle. Examples of this phenomenon include depression, migraine headaches, rheumatoid arthritis, chronic bronchitis, ulcerative colitis, asthma, peptic ulcer, and glaucoma.

There are many diseases not considered to be PMS which are *affected by* PMS. Usually, if your PMS is properly treated, you will at least diminish or eliminate the worsening of symptoms you've been experiencing in the days before you menstruate.

Let's look at some of the conditions that frequently create confusion.

1. *Depression.* (See chapter 5.) You could be suffering from a biochemical depression that peaks during the premenstrual period. Or the stress resulting from difficulties in your life may be causing a situational depression. If you have some degree of depression during the weeks *after* as well as before menstruation, then you need to seek psychological counseling. Though PMS may be part of your problem, it's clearly not the whole problem.

2. *Fatigue and lethargy.* We're all tired some of the time, and there are so many physical and psychological reasons for being tired that fatigue is one of the most difficult conditions to diagnose correctly. If you feel that your fatigue extends throughout the month, then check out some possibilities in addition to PMS. Look into:

   a. **Hypothyroidism.** Thyroid dysfunction causes severe fatigue. For a complete discussion of this condition, its symptoms, its treatment, see chapter 21.

   b. **Chronic Fatigue Syndrome.** CFS is a real condition, probably caused by a virus acting in combination with other immune depressing conditions such as poor diet, yeast infections, intestinal parasites, and other infections. For more information see chapter 21.

   c. **Yeast Infections**. Yeast infections—caused by the *Candida albicans* yeast that is a normal part of the bacteria flora of the human intestinal tract—can cause far more widespread and serious problems than most physicians realize. Certainly, they can cause an overwhelming fatigue. See chapter 21 for a fuller discussion.

Four Different Ways PMS Acts to Produce Symptoms

Psychological ways:

Anxiety
Depresssion
Hypoglycemia
Irritability
Lethargy
Obsessive compulsive
   behaviors
Tension

Water Retention:

Bloatedness (abdominal)
Backache
Dizziness or vertigo
Edema (leg swelling)
Joint pain
Visual disturbance
Weight gain

Allergic responses:

Asthma
Runny or stuffed nose
Skin eruptions or rashes

Lowered resistance
to infection:

Upper respiratory
   infections
Acne
Conjunctivitis
   (reddening of eye lining)

3. *Headaches.* Headaches have many complex causes. It's entirely possible that for some portion of your life headaches—especially migraines—may be part of your destiny, alleviated but not cured by treatment. But our experience is that they can usually be helped, especially if they are worse during your premenstrual days. The next chapter discusses

hypoglycemia and it could be that by studying it you'll learn how to lessen or even abolish your headaches during the entire month.

4. *Food cravings and compulsive eating.* You've probably seen these disturbing symptoms increase during your premenstrual days. If you suffer from them during the rest of the month, then watch out! There are a number of factors that might explain your problem.

   For instance, excessive dieting could be putting you into a very difficult and dangerous relationship to food. Or you might have psychological problems relating to food. We're talking about serious psychiatric disorders like bulimia and anorexia nervosa, which can be lethal.

5. Breast tenderness. You may have high levels of prolactin, the hormone that stimulates the secretion of milk in the breasts.

6. Bloatedness. (See the Interlude in Part III for information on fluid retention.)

Some Degree of PMS

Having said all of the above, remember our first principle: if you have symptoms exclusively or primarily in the premenstrual portion of your month, you have PMS. The corrolary to this is: If you show any increase in well-established, month-long symptoms during the premenstrual period then your condition is presumably being aggravated by *some degree of PMS.*

Do these symptoms occur

a. Only premenstrually?

b. More premenstrually but also postmenstrually (in days 3 to 10 of your cycle), though less frequently postmenstrually?

c. Equally premenstrually and postmenstrually?

d. More postmenstrually?

Now list your symptoms and rate them on a scale of 0 to 10, where 0 represents intense manifestations and 10 indicates the mildest of symptoms.

Symptom   Intensity

_____   _____

_____   _____

_____   _____

Now list all the symptoms for which you have been medically treated and next to the symptom list the treatment.

Symptom   Treatment

_____   _____

_____   _____

_____   _____

As in the case of Clare, you may well find that your treatment has been part of your problem.

4

Fueling Your Brain

THIS CHAPTER WILL SHOW YOU:

- The one critical factor underlying PMS symptoms
- The only substance that keeps your brain running
- Fueling your brain; how it affects your mental symptoms
- How food influences brain functioning
- Why progesterone is crucial to brain functioning
- The first basic steps in beginning to control the problem

To truly understand PMS, you have to fully appreciate the extent to which your brain controls your body. The human brain is an incredibly complex instrument. We are only on the threshold of beginning to comprehend the intricacies of how it works, but we do know that there are certain brain hormones that affect your body, and these can create the changes that you experience as PMS symptoms.

These hormonal changes in the brain are closely related to female sex hormones, particularly estrogen and progesterone, which are connected back to your brain via an intricate *feedback loop.*

Let's look at how symptoms are produced premenstrually. Your brain is the most fuel-demanding organ in your body. It runs only on *glucose* and uses fully twelve percent of the glucose that you ingest to keep itself running.

Any disruption of this fuel supply, no matter how temporary, immediately interferes with your ability to function and may produce the most common PMS symptoms—the psychological/emotional ones: irritability, rage, depression, tension, anxiety, confusion, fatigue, and memory loss.

If there is one single factor that is the key to understanding PMS, it is low blood sugar, or hypoglycemia. If your blood sugar falls too low, then you will be suffering, and if you have the hormonal changes of PMS as well, then this will be bad news for you both emotionally and physically.

The symptoms might be subtle. For instance, minor irritability, frequent fatigue, and annoying, inexplicable food cravings. But, the symptoms could also be really terrible. Intense, "off-the-wall" irritability; wild uncontrollable mood swings that are not predictable to you or anyone else around you; and rage, sometimes hot enough to make even your loved ones flee you as fast as their legs can carry them.

There are other mental dysfunctional states that low blood sugar creates. Memory lapses, inability to concentrate, massive mental fatigue. Worst of all is depression. Some women in their premenstruum fall into a state of severe, even suicidal, depression. In 1956, the MacKinnons, a husband and wife team of doctors, showed that most successful female suicides occurred during the premenstruum. Studies in London, New Delhi, and Los Angeles have confirmed that half of all women's suicide attempts were made during the four days before or the four days after monthly menstruation begins.

What this range of symptoms, from mild to mortal, have in common is that they're related to the inadequate functioning of the brain. That intricately constructed and highly effective mental apparatus is suffering the equivalent of an electrical brownout. It needs more fuel. And it needs that fuel delivered reliably.

What Can Low Blood Sugar Do to You?

As we have seen, low blood sugar can produce a variety of effects, but the story of one young woman is worth a thousand abstract explanations.

Karen M., at twenty-eight, was already a successful editor at a New York publishing house. She was a person who had always been conspicuous for her straightforward positive attitude and her high energy level. More and more frequently, however, during the two weeks prior to her period, those qualities were precisely the ones she couldn't seem to count on. She would become very tense as the day wore on, and by the late afternoon, the tension turned into irritability. She would often have a headache at the same time and, for an hour or two at the end of the work day, would feel washed out and exhausted. For several days, she snapped at people and then in the last day or so before her period, the tension would peak. Rational Karen, always cool and poised, became raging Karen.

One day at an afternoon editorial meeting, she completely lost control, shouting at one of the senior editors. When she looked around and saw that everyone was staring at her, Karen burst into tears and left the room. Years later, she told me she thought that single incident had cost her a year or two in her career.

How could someone so energetic and determined fall apart so completely once a month? The answer lies in the fact that every month, premenstrually, Karen was working with a crippled brain. She didn't act like the same person because she wasn't really the same person. A Rolls Royce that's given some poorly designed synthetic fuel isn't the same car as it is when it's given high octane gasoline. Karen's fatigue, her anger, her catastrophic mood swings were simply the result of her desperate attempts to cope with an energy-deprived brain starved of glucose.

What Causes Low Blood Sugar?

You are what you eat. In fact you are *what* and *when* you eat. In Karen's case, the pressures of her job had habituated her to a very haphazard eating schedule that often included little or no lunch. Once she began consuming frequent small meals and never going more than three hours without eating, her symptoms disappeared almost entirely.

Anyone can have low blood sugar. It doesn't happen because there isn't enough sugar in your diet, but paradoxically, because there is too much. Very briefly, let's look at how your nutritional intake works to fuel your brain.

The food you eat is converted into blood sugar (glucose) and other needed nutrients. After a meal the glucose level rises. In succeeding hours, it slowly drifts back down to a level at which it needs replenishment, or, if food is not available, your body will tap into its stored glycogen.

When you eat your body absorbs certain substances from your foods, mostly through the surface of your small intestine. From carbohydrates, your body absorbs simple sugars, which are, or quickly become, glucose. From fats, it takes glycerol and fatty acids. From proteins, it absorbs amino acids, the building blocks of protein. Variable percentages of the glycerol, fatty acids, and amino acids you absorb from fat and protein are convertible to glucose, thus serving part of your immediate brain energy needs.

Since your body uses glucose for fuel, it might seem sensible to eat as much carbohydrate as possible so as to obtain that fuel most directly. Unfortunately, it's not that simple. If the carbohydrate you eat is the overrefined carbohydrate so common in the modern world—the carbohydrate of table sugar, alcohol, high fructose corn syrup, white flour, or concentrates like fruit juices—then you would be making a fundamental mistake.

The trouble with these *simple* carbohydrates, (as opposed to the *complex* carbohydrates found in vegetables, fruits, and starches) is that they overload the system with glucose. Our bodies, after all, were designed many millennia ago, long before refined carbohydrates were available. When you eat simple carbohydrates, your body overreacts and you actually end up with too little sugar. Even real fruit juices, when used excessively, can cause a problem because they are too concentrated a form of fructose.

Your body controls your blood glucose levels with the help of *insulin*, a truly crucial hormone, best known because the lack of it causes diabetes. After a meal, as your glucose levels go up, insulin is secreted to lower them, because too much glucose is also harmful. However, if the food you eat raises your blood glucose level very rapidly, then insulin will overreact and lower that level very sharply indeed. That's the crucial paradox. The net result of eating the wrong foods is a blood glucose level *lower* than it was before you ate.

That's why such foods as a glass of wine, a candy bar, or an ice cream cone, after an initial burst of energy, produce an unpleasant energy crash. A vigorous outrush of insulin, responding to what it sees as a dangerous sugar overload, has sent your glucose level plummeting. But that isn't the end of the story. Your body has techniques for dealing with almost any problem. When your glucose levels get knocked too far down by an outrush of insulin, your body promptly releases *counterregulatory hormones*—glucagon, adrenocorticoids, and adrenalin—to raise the glucose level back up.

Adrenalin causes the liver to send glucose directly into the bloodstream, particularly following long intervals (more than three hours) between meals or snacks. It's the hormone that sets the body's "fight-or-flight" mechanism in motion; it causes an increased heart rate, increased blood pressure, and a shift in the mental state toward increased neuronal excitability. Many women find that a release of adrenalin causes nervousness, irritability, panic attack, or migraine headaches. Under the influence of sudden surges of adrenalin, you may start feeling faint, shaky, and weak, or even experience heart palpitations.

You can see that nutrition involves far more than just getting your vitamins. Controlling Premenstrual Syndrome is first and foremost a matter of controlling the food you eat and the liquid you drink, so that your brain will be adequately fueled.

The Progesterone Connection

In the last chapter, you saw that a relative shortage of progesterone is the pivotal causational factor in Premenstrual Syndrome. All the precipitating factors noted—including pregnancies, abortions, miscarriages, tubal ligations, oral contraceptives, hysterectomies, and simply aging—can contribute to progesterone deficit. One way that this relative lack of progesterone affects you is by aggravating the fuel crisis that eating the wrong foods tends to cause.

It has been found that because of the hormonal changes in the premenstruum, a woman's body becomes more sensitized to drops in blood sugar at that time. The same decrease in blood sugar that produces only minor discomfort *after* menstruation may produce a devastating reaction before menstruation.

This is what commonly happens to women with PMS. *The major factors in most cases of PMS are this blood sugar drop and its consequences.* Keep that fact firmly in mind, and you will understand most of your PMS problem. The chapters in the second part of this book will make a good deal of sense, and you will be able to use the treatment plan effectively.

And what about the progesterone connection? Does this mean you'll have to take progesterone to control your low blood sugar response? In most cases, no! The right diet can control the problem quite satisfactorily 75 percent of the time. If diet alone doesn't work, then we do turn to natural progesterone. The only way to find out if it's needed is to optimize your diet. We'll show you how to do that, and those of you for whom it's not sufficient will find that chapter 18 clearly explains the ins and outs of progesterone therapy.

Our nutrition section (chapter 15) will show you the type of diet that works, but for now let's look at some of the guiding principles that will keep your blood sugar from falling too low.

Controlling Your Brain's Fuel Supply

There are clear steps you can take to avoid low blood sugar.

1. *Avoid problem foods.* It's particularly important to avoid forms of sugar such as alcohol, citrus juice, and simple sugar itself. You may have cravings for candy bars. Part of the process of controlling your PMS will be preventing or controlling those cravings during the premenstrual portion of each month. The foods you should be eating during the

CLINICAL CLUES

Testing yourself: Do You Have Low Blood Sugar?

- After you go too long without eating do you get dizzy? Lose your concentration? Become irritable? Feel tired, weak, or even depressed?
- Do you wake up in the middle of the night with either panic or anxiety attacks?
- Do you crave candy bars?
- Do you feel tired after eating a heavy meal?
- Do you feel more fatigued after taking sugar?
- Do certain foods make you tired, irritable, or depressed? Do these foods contain obvious sugar (ice cream, cola drinks) or perhaps hidden sugar like so many "health food" muffins that are on the market?

If you answered "yes" to any of the above questions, you may have a diagnosis of episodic PMS-related low blood sugar.

Here are four suggestions that may help you:
- Make a list of the foods you like and can eat without problems.
- Make a list of the foods that make you tired.
- Make a list of the foods that make you irritable or depressed.
- Keep available and use only the foods that don't create problems.

premenstruum are complex carbohydrates and high protein foods because they will best provide a prolonged and steady energy supply for your brain. Once you've got a craving, you're already in the downward spiral of low blood sugar. It's much easier to prevent cravings than to struggle to control them.

2. *Don't go too long without eating!* Teach yourself to eat frequent small meals. Many women find that eating small amounts every two or three hours is effective. Some small complex carbohydrate or protein snack strategically situated halfway between breakfast and lunch, lunch and dinner, and before bed may be just the thing to keep your blood glucose level on an even keel.

3. *Adjust volume of food to activity level.* If you have an early dinner and afterward engage in physical activity, follow that activity with a high protein or complex carbohydrate snack. If you find yourself waking up in the morning with a headache, then have a late night snack before you go to bed. Remember when you're sleeping, you're fasting.

Foods to Consider with Caution

Dawn was a certified nutritionist. She probably knew more about many areas of nutrition than we did, and she was willing to accept the news that she was being affected by recurrent shortages of fuel to the brain. So why didn't she get better?

It turned out that Dawn started each day with a glass of "nutritious" freshly squeezed orange juice. This simple sugar drove her blood sugar straight up. Then insulin overreacted and drove her blood sugar straight down. Like most people she had been deceived by misleading advertising. While the vitamin C in orange juice is very healthy, the high level of natural sugar contained in the juice is terrible for PMS sufferers.

If you're suffering the symptoms of low blood sugar, you'll have to be careful of sugar in all its forms. Avoid maltose, dextrose, fructose, glucose, corn syrup, and even the natural sugar in citrus juices. Every year, we "cure" a dozen or more severe sufferers of PMS simply by convincing them to eliminate citrus juice from their diet.

Simple sugars may be found in some of your favorite foods, both healthful and unhealthful. *Ketchup is almost 50 percent sugar!*

Perhaps more surprisingly, most of these luscious bran muffins that have been so misleadingly marketed as "healthy" snacks are prepared with concentrated fruit juices and are therefore loaded with sugar. You'll find that most baked goods contain sugar in some form. Also avoid products containing carob. Stay away from soft drinks and also be wary of "training" drinks like Gatorade®. Even some fruits should be eaten in moderation during your premenstrual days. Raisins and grapes frequently cause too rapid a rise in blood sugar and citrus fruits require caution. One orange may not harm you—unless you're very sensitive—because its juice is packaged in its natural cellulose lining and that slows the distribution of sugar, but two oranges or more could well bring on all the dreaded hypoglycemic symptoms.

Are You Sure You're Suffering Premenstrually from Low Blood Sugar?

If premenstrually, you have the symptoms we've been talking about, there really is very little doubt that you suffer from the effects of low blood sugar. But if there is any uncertainty, consider having a Glucose Tolerance Test (GTT). It is crucial to have this test in the premenstrual period, (when you are having symptoms), so you can find out how your body responds to being challenged by sugar. *The most important aspect of a GTT is timing.* Blood sugar levels are closely related to levels of body and brain hormones, particularly progesterone.

A GTT is called a provocative test, one that essentially provokes your body to do its worst. That means the test is a bit of an ordeal. You have to fast from midnight the night before, then go to a laboratory where a baseline sample of blood is taken. Next you swallow a thick sugary drink, and then have blood drawn once an hour for four to six hours. The test can be stressful, requiring time, effort, and increased fatigue, so most women simply don't go and get tested when they should—which is premenstrually, at the time of the month when they're feeling absolutely terrible. If you go premenstrually, then your blood sugar curve will show your hypoglycemic abnormality. But, when you're not premenstrual, it most likely will not, and the test will have been wasted.

But there is another problem: Most doctors don't read these tests very precisely because they're not attuned to the difference between *dynamic* and *static* tests. The GTT is a dynamic test; it measures the *rate of change* as well as providing absolute numbers. A cursory glance at just the high and low numbers will not lead to an accurate assessment of what is going wrong, and far too many physicians look at the numbers that way.

But, if you have Premenstrual Syndrome, it's going to be one of the most useful tests you'll ever take. In chapter 19 we'll give you a detailed explanation of how you can interpret your own Glucose Tolerance Test.

In closing this chapter we want to reiterate that low blood sugar plays a role in an exceedingly wide range of premenstrual symptoms. Once you find how to assure a steady delivery of the right fuel to your body and thus to your brain, you may find that PMS itself is under control.

We hope you now have a firm sense of the basics. In Part II, you will begin to learn more about what we call the masks of PMS— the conditions that are most often misdiagnosed upon presentation of PMS symptoms. We hope you've never been misdiagnosed as seriously as the women you'll meet in Part II, but we know there's a fair chance you have been.

Interlude

Six Helpful Hints for Better Sleep

Proper sleep is important to maintaining the natural biochemical basis of your body, yet it is often difficult to obtain in an over-stressed life. Sleep is not something you can take for granted. Don't assume that whatever you're getting is just going to have to be enough. If you're not getting enough restful, restorative sleep, you aren't going to feel too well.

Women often find that their sleep is more disturbed premenstrually. This can be because of increased tension and irritability, or it can be caused by your blood sugar level plummeting during the middle of the night. If that occurs, it will, of course, send your brain fuel down to precariously low levels.

Of course, there can be a thousand reasons—anything from travel or other alterations in your familiar environment to illness or the introduction of children into your life—for irregularities in your nightly rest. As your own therapist, it's your responsibility to work out a plan that will insure you a good night's sleep.

Here are five things that can help:

1. Eat a specially designed snack at bedtime. This should include serotonin-providing foods such as cheese, bananas, or milk. Eat a small amount of protein at the same time. Forget the notion that you shouldn't eat at bedtime, but be careful not to eat to much or your abdomen will become distended. And be cautious about milk. If you have a lactose intolerance then it can be more of a hindrance than a help.

2. Make sure you aren't taking in any hidden sources of caffeine. That will require diligently reading labels. Many diet drinks include caffeine to replace the sugar "high" of regular soda. This can be habit forming. You should limit your consumption to one early morning cup of coffee.

3. Do ten minutes of stretching exercises right before bedtime. Our muscles need to become deeply relaxed when we sleep, and a stretching program can prepare you for sleep even before your head hits the pillow.

   Don't do any aerobic exercise in the late evening. Such an exercise is certainly great for your health, but done just before bedtime, it tends to keep people awake. It causes significant altering changes in the brain biochemistry. On the other hand, twenty-five minutes of aerobic exercise in the morning is a splendid way to energize your day.

4. Don't be afraid to hire a sleep consultant. If you have chronic insomnia, work with a doctor to see whether the *short-term* use of the medications might be valuable in changing your sleep patterns. The use of mild tranquilizers with a short half-life (that is, ones that do not linger in your body) can often help to initiate that change. Our preference among mild tranquilizers are Ativan® or Serax®, because they have few side effects.

5. Learn some relaxation exercises or take up yoga. You might purchase one of the many effective audio tapes to help induce sleep. Such tapes can also be extraordinarily useful in relaxing your muscles.

MASKS AND MISDIAGNOSES

5

PMS Depression

- How PMS is very commonly misdiagnosed as depression
- How drug mistreatment often follows
- That PMS depression is generally related to low blood sugar
- How to use your menstrual calendar to establish a proper diagnosis

How can you help me? I've done everything already, and nobody seems to know the answer. I've seen three gynecologists, an endocrinologist, a therapist, and even a psychiatrist for medicines, and nothing has helped. Oh well, some things helped for a little while . . . the Pill . . . Elavil® . . . even Xanax®, though it made me awfully sleepy. But then my depression just got worse and worse. I don't know why I'm here.

The speaker is our patient, Caroline D., a thirty-four-year-old real estate broker with PMS. She was speaking for countless women who came into our center dragging behind them a long trail of PMS misdiagnosed as depression. Over and over again, major studies show more women are depressed than men. Seldom is it even considered that the explanation for that difference might be PMS.

Sixty percent of our PMS patients come to us having received diagnosis and/or treatment for depression at some time. Depression is probably the most damaging misdiagnosis we encounter. We see women treated for years without improvement while their lives are wasted. But a diagnosis of premenstrual depression is usually easy to establish if you look for it in the proper way.

When we started PMS Medical, our center in Manhattan in 1979, we imagined that women would come to us by very varied paths, and they did. But after a while, we began to see that patients divided into two main types. The first were intelligent, media-informed women who had had to make the correct diagnosis all by themselves, because there wasn't any real medical help available. Magazine articles, television reporting, or word-of-mouth pointed them in the right direction. The second type was more distressing. These women had gone through a maze of doctors—sometimes more than a dozen. By the time they came to us, their faith in medicine was feeble at best.

In 1984, we did a study of twenty-five consecutive admissions to our PMS Center. These women averaged five previous physicians and bills of $4,750. Their treatments had resulted in little or no improvement. It was an embarrassing commentary on the relationship between PMS and American medicine.

This chapter will show you how you can ascertain whether you have PMS or one of the various forms of depression—or both. We'll be laying the groundwork in this chapter, so that further on you'll be able to use the same guidelines to rule out other frequent misdiagnoses.

The Great Escape: How Karla Eluded Her Misdiagnosis

Karla J., thirty-one, appeared like a waif washed up at our office door. Incredibly she had just escaped from a psychiatric unit in one of New York's most prestigious hospitals. She'd been receiving treatment for severe depression with suicidal intent.

The week before our unscheduled meeting, Karla, a paralegal, had swallowed an overdose of sleeping pills and was taken by ambulance to the hospital emergency room. She was placed in a locked ward because her history showed two previous suicide attempts. In the course of ten years of severe depressions, Karla had received numerous treatments with different antidepressants, including Elavil®, and Tofranil®. After several meetings, the staff at the prestigious hospital came to the conclusion that Karla needed the last resort for unmanageable depression—electroshock therapy.

After three treatments her depression started to improve, although she was experiencing memory loss, a common result of electroshock. Nonetheless, she appeared to be getting better. The staff felt relieved and began to congratulate themselves on their wisdom. (Though they had failed to notice that Karla had started to menstruate; a fact which—as this whole book is designed to demonstrate—can have diagnostic significance.) Taking no chances, the physicians decided they would go ahead with more electroshock.

Shortly after the third treatment, Karla was sitting in the dayroom listening to the radio. Dr. Martorano was being interviewed on a local talk show, and the subject was PMS. Midway through the interview, Karla jumped up and yelled to the nurses to come and listen.

"I don't think I'm just depressed," Karla announced to them, like someone who has seen the light. *"I have Premenstrual Syndrome."*

The nurses tried not to laugh. Karla insisted on speaking to her physician, and the resident went over her case with her briefly, then dismissed her new insight with the blanket comment that he didn't believe in PMS. Maybe, after she finished the shock treatments, she would be well enough to enter some more sustained form of psychoanalysis.

That afternoon Karla escaped from the hospital, looked up our address in the phone book, walked forty blocks in the rain to our office, and sat herself down, dripping wet, in our waiting room until we could squeeze her in for a consultation.

Her story, though unusual, is not unique. Do we need to tell you that Karla was absolutely right in her self-diagnosis? Can you, in your wildest dreams, imagine having to flee a respected hospital to get the right treatment?

Another, More Complex Story

Jane A., thirty-eight, was a housewife who had had episodes of depression since she was twenty-one. She began seeing a social worker for psychotherapy when she was twenty-three, but her periods of depression persisted and worsened at times.

When she was twenty-five, Jane became engaged. She thought she would get better once she married, and, in spite of a rocky engagement and a terrible honeymoon, it seemed at first that this might happen.

Jane was very happy in her marriage. When she wasn't suffering for PMS, she was delightful—a warm, lovely person whom her husband adored. Unfortunately, the good times became less frequent. Jane was depressed more and more frequently, and the length of her depression increased. The couple decided to have children, hoping that Jane would feel better. But, after each of her pregnancies, her condition became noticeably worse. After the second child she was diagnosed as having *postpartum depression*. (In all probability she did—most postpartum depression is related to PMS.)

NOTHING WAS HELPING

> When I got depressed I was so sad, so tired, absolutely unable to do anything. All I wanted to do was crawl into bed with the covers over my head. Al, my husband, was horrified. The more he tried to help me, the worse it became. I couldn't even take care of my own children and that made me feel even worse about myself!

Jane was still seeing the same social worker she began with, and the therapist very sensibly (though belatedly) referred her to a psychiatrist, Dr. P. She was showing clear signs of suicidal preoccupation.

The psychiatrist prescribed a half milligram of Xanax®, a tranquilizer which, incidentally, has been touted as being useful in PMS. Jane took the pill three times a day *and fell asleep three times a day.* Frustrated, Dr. P. decided to give Jane an antidepressant. He chose Elavil®, which—until Prozac® became available—was the most commonly used antidepressant. There was a slight improvement and then a regression in which the symptoms got even worse.

Not understanding the connection between Jane's depression and her menstrual cycle, Dr. P. increased the dose more and more for three months while Jane continued to suffer from her cyclical depression.

MORE HELP, MORE DISORDER

When Dr. P. saw that the increased dosage wasn't working, he was concerned, and he switched to another commonly used antidepressant, Tofranil®, 25 mgs., three times a day. The same thing happened! Jane seemed to get better for a little while and then mysteriously relapsed.

Finally, Jane's deeply frustrated psychiatrist went the distance, putting her on Nardil®, an MAO inhibitor[1]. This is a dangerous class of drugs with numerous side effects, including a potentially lethal interaction with a number of common foods such as aged cheese and wine.

UNDERSTANDING WHAT HAPPENED

Figure 1 shows the pattern of false assumptions that deceived both the psychiatrist and the social worker. First they made the assumption that Jane had a depressive reaction and treated it with psychotherapy.

When this didn't work they then assumed poor Jane had a biochemical depression and started using antidepressants. Now note a very interesting phenomenon that we commonly observe. Since women with PMS are most depressed premenstrually, that is when the antidepressant is usually started or the dosage is

---

[1] An MAO inhibitor is a drug that prevents the activity of the enzyme monoamine oxidase (MAO) in the brain and therefore affects the moods.

increased. An antidepressant usually takes ten days to two weeks to become effective. *By this time, the patient has started menstruating, and there is a marked lessening of the depressive symptoms of PMS anyway.*

Eureka! The doctor almost always erroneously attributes the patient's improvement to the antidepressant. But he hardly has time to finish congratulating himself when the woman starts the PMS phase of her cycle again. He concludes that now his drug is no longer working, since her depression begins worsening once more.

The physician is puzzled. Perhaps he has been too timid. He increases the dose. The same pattern repeats itself. Always he is seduced by the improvement in the postmenstruum. The drugs seem effective initially, and then suddenly a moment arrives when they no longer appear to be working. (The physician with four years of medical school and four years of postgraduate training in a hospital doesn't understand what you're going to learn simply by superimposing your treatment chart over your menstrual calendar!)

But let's get back to Jane. In addition to treating her with medication, her psychiatrist saw her once a week for psychotherapy. Jane quit three times in disgust, because she didn't seem to be making any progress but, since her married life rocketed back and forth between relative tranquility and sheer Hell, she inevitably came back to therapy. Give the psychiatrist *some* credit. He was probably the anchor that prevented her from committing suicide. His problem was that he simply wasn't treating the right disorder.

At last, after seventeen years of episodic and near-suicidal depression, a better stage in Jane's story began. Sarah, one of her closest friends, also suffered from PMS-related depression. She told Jane she thought she would come to our Center for an evaluation. In fact, she even called and made the appointment for Jane.

When Jane came in, we found that her PMS depression (as well as most of her other PMS symptoms, including breast tenderness and bloating) peaked at ovulation, then declined, then went up again in the week before her menstrual flow. This is one of the common types of PMS. Her blood sugar levels were the first thing we looked at.

Figure 1. Is the Antidepressant Working?

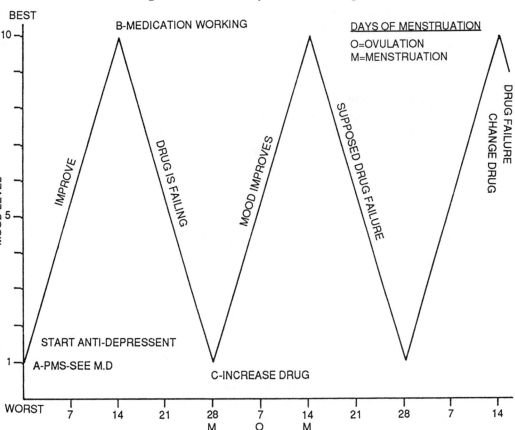

A physician convinced a patient is depressed generally tries the antidepressant drugs sooner or later.

In this graph, the mood level goes up and down, apparently in response to the administration of a drug that has initial good effects but then begins to fail. Actually the changes are in response to PMS. The drug was given when the patient was in the depths of PMS-induced depression. The patient then improved naturally in the course of the next seven to ten days. (Coincidentally this is the time it takes for an antidepressant to start working.)

If an antidepressant had actually been the cause of improvement, then after the graph shot up (a minimum gain of + 3 on the mood scale), the graph would have shown a more or less stable plateau throughout the month with no further gigantic dips or rises.

We put Jane on an appropriate diet. She soon showed a *50 percent* improvement, but her depressions were so severe that this was not enough, so we gave her natural progesterone twice a day. In a very short time, her depression was gone, and it has not returned. She has the energy to care for her children. Both her kids and her husband can count on her, now.

Jane continued to take progesterone for five months. We then took her off it and she was able to continue simply with a nutritional plan that prevented hypoglycemic fall in blood sugar during the premenstrual half of each month. She has had no therapeutic intervention. We see her once a year, and she tells us that her depression is a thing of the past. Just a bad, old memory.

Do 60 Percent of Women with PMS Also Have Depression?

More women with PMS are misdiagnosed as *depressives* than any other form of misdiagnosis. We see women who have been treated for depression with tranquilizers, with antidepressant, with analysis—and, like Karla, even with electroshock therapy. All without sustained improvement!

Yet *PMS depression* is almost always ignored by the medical establishment. Reported surveys of depression clearly indicate that women experience far more depression than men. Given the occurrence rate of PMS and the frequency with which it manifests itself as depression, we're convinced that the higher statistical frequency of depression in women is almost entirely due to PMS.

As we have noted, *60 percent of the patients who come into our center have already been treated for some form of depression.*

There are two major reasons for this high percentage of misdiagnosis. First, most PMS sufferers are depressed. But this doesn't mean they're suffering from "depression." To say someone is depressed, as ordinary people say it in ordinary conversation, is different from a precise medical definition of depression.

You can be depressed as a consequence of serious problems in your life—that's called a *situational depression*. Or you can be depressed as a physical consequence of illness. Or the medications you're taking can depress you. Or you can be *biochemically depressed*—this is the most serious and severe form of depression and in psychiatry is referred to as *chemical depression*. Finally, you can be *hormonally depressed* premenstrually. And that's PMS. This depression is related to a *hypoglycemic* response (a lowering of your blood sugar) premenstrually. Hypoglycemia is a Greek word derived from *hypo* meaning "under," *glykis* meaning "sweet," and *emia* "meaning "in the blood." Consequently it means *too little sugar in the blood.*

There is a lot of confusion and controversy over this particular medical term. Many physicians use it interchangeably with low blood sugar. Other physicians, however, raise their eyebrows at the very mention of the word. This is probably because they confuse *reactive hypoglycemia* with *medical hypoglycemia*. Reactive hypoglycemia is the name for the type of low blood sugar we described in chapter 4. It's not a steady state of low blood sugar but rather frequent, rapid, inappropriate drops in blood sugar levels. Medical hypoglycemia, on the other hand, refers to certain relatively rare and dangerous conditions in which the blood sugar falls to a low level and essentially stays there.

As you recall your brain runs on glucose (blood sugar). There's nothing else that fuels your brain, and, if not enough glucose is available in your bloodstream, your brain won't run at its optimal level, and you'll experience this as depression, confusion, or cognitive "brown out."

Not only are there several types of depression, but you also can have more than one type of depressive condition simultaneously. No wonder your doctors have been confused!

The second reason for so much misdiagnosis of PMS is that physicians diagnose according to their training, and their training has generally not included any great discussion of Premenstrual Syndrome. And, in the diagnostic swamp of PMS-related depression, it isn't just doctors who'll be trying out their particular conviction on you. Social workers, psychologists, and ministers functioning as psychotherapists—they're all eager to treat a hormonal disorder with talk or even, heaven help us, with massages, meditation, or group therapy. Might be good for you, but hardly for your PMS.

You should also remember that too many doctors have had training that includes almost no mention of reactive hypoglycemia. A good way to check out your physician is to ask him his feelings about hypoglycemia. If he believes in it, and knows about glucose tolerance tests, and understands that a diet high in sugar and refined carbohydrates can actually push your blood sugar levels down, then you're on a sound footing.

However, if he tells you "I don't believe in hypoglycemia," then you ought to look elsewhere. He probably hasn't thought about low blood sugar since he read the one required paragraph on it in medical school.

One patient of ours, Marie, persuaded her doctor to give her a Glucose Tolerance Test, and when the test caused a severe drop in her blood sugar levels, she actually fainted in his office. "She's a nervous type," her doctor said dismissively. None so deaf, as those that will not hear.

If you suffer from depression and you want to determine how closely related it is to your menstrual cycle, just move on to the next section of this chapter.

Use Your Menstrual Calendar to Calculate Your Depression

Look at your menstrual calendar. If your mood averages under 5 on our mood rating scale, you are probably suffering from some sort of depression.

If your low numbers occur only in the premenstrual part of your cycle you probably have PMS. (See Figure 2.) It's important to note your mood several times a day because PMS-related depression, being largely related to changes in your blood sugar levels, often fluctuates throughout the day. There are more mood changes in PMS depression than in any other forms of depression.

Figure 2.

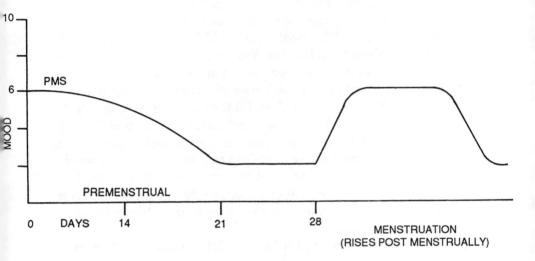

In PMS your mood scale may drop premenstrually and return to an average level of 6.5 or more on days 3 to 7 postmenstrually, averaging a gain of 4 to 5 points on you mood scale. This is clearly a graph for PMS rather than depression.

Let's say you came up with an average of 3 for the *entire month*. Now find the average for your postmenstrual period. If that postmenstrual number is three points or more above the average for the entire month, then you probably have a diagnosis of PMS.

If we were your clinician, we would recommend a Glucose Tolerance Test (GTT), premenstrually, to see if your blood sugar is being adversely affected by your hormonal changes. In short, you would find out if you're experiencing a premenstrual drop in blood sugar.

But if your low numbers also occur postmenstrually, as in Figure 3—then you have some other form of depression. It could be biochemical or situational, or it could be a month-long condition of hypoglycemia related to your diet.

The numbers you record on your menstrual calendar will help you to decide what's going on. We have seen women who averaged 2.0 during the premenstrual and 3.0 during the postmenstrual period. Clearly PMS had only a *minor* part to play in their depression. Sometimes by an appropriate diet alone such a patient has improved to a reasonable extent—up to 3 or 4 points. We would assume in such a case that what we were treating was largely a depression cause by low blood sugar. In other cases, where there was virtually no change, we would look for a biochemical or situational depression.

Now before you go any further, carefully examine the two-week period before you start menstruating. (See Figure 4.) If your overall monthly average is low and you find there is a further dip right before your period, you may have a combination of biochemical depression with PMS depression.

We have learned from experience that in such cases, we treat the PMS first. Then, if depression persists, we re-evaluate the situation.

Your numbers may show that you may have a month-long depression. What you'll see on your menstrual calendar is more variation in your mood than normal on a daily basis. If you have such daily dips in your blood sugar levels, what you have or haven't eaten is constantly affecting your mood level throughout the day.

We've seen many patients who fit this description. Usually they are among the most elusive of the depressives. Many have gone from doctor to doctor. The most severe have utterly brutalized

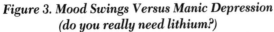

*Figure 3. Mood Swings Versus Manic Depression
(do you really need lithium?)*

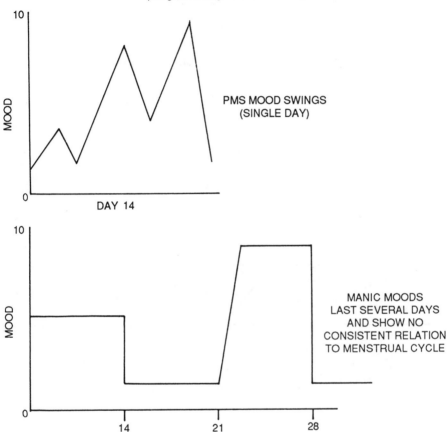

Manic depression is relentlessly overdiagnosed and confused with mood swings. Most mood swings seem to be more related to underlying hormonal imbalances such as those reflected by changes in your low blood sugar.

To separate out manic depressive disease from PMS related mood swings, the commonest cause of misdiagnosis, rate your mood several times a day.

If your mood fluctuates several times within a twenty-four hour period, it is unlikely you have manic depression. To establish if the mood swing are due to PMS compare the moods pre- and post-menstrually. If the mood swings are basically limited to the pre-menstrual period, you probably have PMS.

Figure 4. Depression Exacerbated by PMS

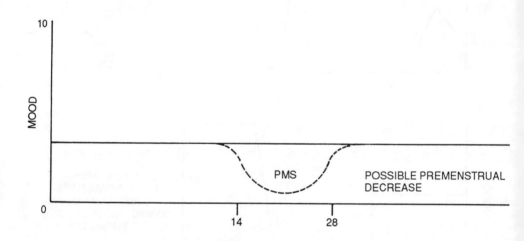

In depression your mood doesn't rise significantly postmenstru-ally, although there may be some additional drop premenstrually (if there is a premenstrual aspect to your depression).

lives. The great majority, even with moderate to mild hypogly-cemia, are baffled by a life they can't seem to control. Marie, the patient who fainted in her doctor's office, had been treated for depression for fourteen years. When we asked her about it, she said with brief and bitter eloquence, "I'm *always* depressed." Her depression turned out to be entirely related to the fact that her brain wasn't getting enough fuel.

Look for PMS First

The bottom line in this discussion is that *unless it's clear from your menstrual calendar that there's no connection between your de-pression and your monthly cycle, you should be taking care of your PMS first.* Once you've done that you will probably find your depression has dissipated or even vanished. Of course, if your depression is extremely severe, then you had best proceed with the help of a physician. Just try to make sure that he or she is also knowledgeable about PMS and considers it in your differential diagnosis.

6

Mood Swings and Manic Depression

THIS CHAPTER WILL SHOW YOU:

- How PMS-induced mood swings can be taken for manic depression and other psychiatric "cycling" disorders
- The dangers inherent in such a misdiagnosis
- How to avoid misdiagnosis
- Not taking lithium lightly
- What to do if you do have manic depressive disorder and PMS

Mood swings are among the most difficult symptoms to diagnose. Certainly most of us have normal mood swings ranging from elation to dejection and, on very somber occasions, perhaps even despair. However, frequent and extreme mood swings can lead to severe difficulties. They are hard to diagnose and even harder to treat. Only too often the patient with prolonged elation feels "too good" to be treated, and the despairing patient feels "too bad" to keep her appointment.

If this is true of mood swings, it is doubly true of manic depressive disorder, a far more serious and biologically different illness that can, however, bear a striking similarity to severe mood swings when looked at by the untrained eye of a lay person.

Advances Have Led to More Complications

In recent years there have emerged a number of highly effective drugs for the treatment of specific psychiatric diseases. The one involving mood swings and manic depression that you have probably heard the most about is lithium. Lithium represents a great advance in medical treatment, especially for manic depression, a genetic disorder characterized by severe changes in mood.

Unfortunately, as these advances were refined, subclassifications of the disease also proliferated. Today there are a number of incredibly confusing diagnoses sprouting like weeds in the psychiatric garden. Even the most sophisticated physician would have trouble dealing with them. As the nomenclature committee of the American Psychiatric Association continues to rewrite and reclassify disorders, even seasoned clinicians are confused by their categories. Terms like "bipolar" and its many children—Bipolar I, Bipolar II, Bipolar III, Rapid Cycling Disorders—have been coined, supposedly to clarify and better define different forms of manic depression. Actually, the situation is muddy, indeed.

Nonetheless, even if there is confusion in terminology and diagnosis, it's very fortunate that we now have drugs that can help with extreme mood swings, including the relatively rare manic depressive disorder. The bad news is that in this climate we see simple mood swings being overdiagnosed as more serious disorders and relentlessly overtreated with dangerous drugs that produce highly questionable results.

There are too many patients on lithium, a great drug when needed, but one with potentially severe side effects. There are also too many patients being treated with crossover drugs from the anti-epileptic arsenal, like Tegretol® and Depakote®. These drugs have been found to be effective in certain severe mood disorders, such as Rapid Cycling Disorder, which produces a sharp emotional plunge—from elation to despair—in patients.

Some of these patients are, of course, being appropriately treated before an appropriate differential diagnosis is established. We contend that this differential diagnosis must include PMS, for many of the women who are being diagnosed this way are actually victims of PMS.

Are You Manic Depressive?

Ordinary mood swings might cause you to think yourself a manic depressive. So let's consider how different ordinary mood swings are from real mania.

The criteria for mania include the presence of three or four of the items listed below for a period of no less than a week:

1. intensely increased activity
2. increased speech; both in rate and intensity
3. ideas flying through your mind at the speed of light
4. inflated self-esteem (grandiosity)
5. decreased hours of sleep
6. distractibility
7. an involvement in high-risk activities, such as periods of frenetic sexuality, risky driving, and prolonged periods of binge spending that tend toward bankruptcy

Having studied those seven items, do you still feel you're a true manic depressive? Let me tell you about a woman who thought she was.

Six Years of Treatment

Janet H. was fine for half of each month, but two weeks before her period, she would begin to have sharp alterations of mood several times a day. On the downswing, she would plummet into deep, suicidal despair.

Before she came to see us, Janet had already been hospitalized three times for manic depressive disorder. She had been on lithium for over six years, but she still wasn't completely better. The lithium had seemed to alleviate her problems slightly, but this only encouraged her doctors to raise her dose for maximal effect. Janet would occasionally lapse into lithium toxicity with severe tremors, diarrhea, and general weakness.

No one had ever asked her why her mood swings had occurred prior to her menstrual period. We assumed that her physicians felt that such severe symptoms had to be due to a "serious" underlying mental condition and not to a relatively simple problem like PMS.

We gave Janet a Glucose Tolerance Test. She had a three-hour blood sugar level of 4, which is low. With that information in hand, we still couldn't tell if she was manic depressive, but we certainly know that there was something wrong with the delivery of fuel to her brain. It was a fairly reasonable supposition that the relative lack of progesterone in her premenstruum was making it impossible for her brain to get enough glucose.

We placed Janet on 300 mgs. of the even-release oral tablet of progesterone twice a day and she improved immediately. In fact, she improved so much we were eventually able to wean her off the lithium and conclude that what we had in Janet was a case of PMS successfully treated by a standard PMS protocol.

Could I Have Both?

Is it possible to have both manic depressive disorder and PMS? Certain patients do. An example of this was Eileen D., an artist, who came to us after a long period of problems she felt were, at least in part, related to her menstrual cycle.

In the late 1970s, when she was in her late thirties, she began to suffer a wide variety of symptoms during her premenstruum, including depression, irritability, difficulty concentrating, insomnia, and swollen and painful breasts. In 1979, her female gynecologist suggested she take vitamin B₆, but was not open to any further treatment because "she felt PMS was anti-feminist."

Eileen turned to other physicians, tried vitamins without much effect, and noticed she was suffering extreme mood swings. In the premenstrual portion of the month, she also experienced severe depression. She found she was having frequent suicidal thoughts.

She struggled through to 1986, getting worse, failing to capitalize on several major career opportunities, and not knowing where to go for help. In that year, she went to see a holistic medical doctor and was diagnosed as having allergies and intestinal parasites. The doctor put her on intravenous vitamin C, which she found improved her mood somewhat, and sent her to a specialist who put her on two powerful drugs to treat her parasites. The drugs caused her to experience enormous emotional instability, which, coming at the height of a difficult premenstrual period, caused a nervous breakdown. Eileen ended up in the psychiatric ward of a major New York hospital for a weekend.

Soon after, Eileen began to work with a psychopharmacologist and came to see us. The psychopharmacologist diagnosed her correctly as having bipolar depression; she was indeed manic depressive. But being an enlightened physician he also said to her, "If you have PMS, it will make everything else worse." We found Eileen did indeed have a serious case of PMS. She was given an antidepressant and lithium to control her manic depression throughout the month, and we altered her diet to control hypoglycemic symptoms and gave her progesterone. The dual therapy was highly effective, and Eileen's problems are now well under control.

More About Mood Swings

Mood swings can range from very minor to quite severe in intensity. First of all, it's important to realize that they can be caused by a wide range of precipitating factors. PMS is one of them. It's important and needs to be taken into account. What needs to be mentioned in the matter of mood swings—and so often isn't—is the relationship between brain functioning and mood. The list of things that can influence brain functioning is long indeed.

For instance, mood swings can be triggered by prolonged sleep deprivation. We have seen patients with severely intensified mood swings caused by travel through time zones. The treatment can be rather simple: restore sleep through a simple sleep-inducing medication taken for several days.

Mood swings can be associated with oral contraceptive use, due to its effect on the balance of estrogen and progesterone. After discontinuing the contraceptive, further treatment can consist of supplementation with vitamin B_6, which has usually been depleted. B_6 is essential for the production of two of the most important brain neurotransmitters, dopamine and serotonin, without which your brain couldn't maintain any mood stabilization. Serotonin depletion has been linked to depression, and many of the newer, more effective antidepressants, such as Prozac®, work by increasing the amount of serotonin that gets to your brain.

When supplementing with vitamin B_6, remember to also take B complex supplements. B_6 alone can disturb the intestinal flora and cause excretion of too much of the other B vitamins.

Of course, we're sure you've already guessed that the hypoglycemic effects of Premenstrual Syndrome will also promote mood swings. An erratic delivery of glucose to your brain causes interruptions in functioning; you may experience highs or lows due to changes in your neuroendocrine system.

FAST FOOD DIETS DON'T HELP

Diets that rely heavily on convenience foods don't help. Too much of the natural sources of B vitamins (not to mention many other nutrients) is lost in food processing and storage. Breads made from refined white flour, polished rices—these foods have been rendered practically useless by the refining processes, and it's very hard to eat this way and get proper quantities of B_6. Less B_6, less neurotransmitters to the brain. Modern civilization with its highly processed foods is sacrificing quality to convenience.

ARE YOUR MOOD SWINGS CAUSED BY PMS?

The normal method of monthly charting will, of course, be the chief indicator of whether your mood swings are PMS-related. Chart your mood several times daily at set times. Give it a rating from 0 (severely depressed) to 10 (feeling fine) and keep these records for several months. Perhaps you'll have to use a scale above 10 if your mood becomes elated or hyperactive.

If your mood changes sharply several times a day, and this increases premenstrually, then the most likely cause is PMS. You should get a GTT done premenstrually and analyze it according to the criteria we'll give you in chapter 19.

Once you've established that PMS has a role in your mood swings, you can take precautions. Be especially careful to avoid alcohol, which is a frequent precipitator of mood swings, and be diligent in avoiding oral contraceptives and other synthetic progestogens.

Another clinical point: Carefully evaluate any medications you may be taking. You will probably need the assistance of your doctor here. Medications like steroids and blood pressure pills are frequently associated with changes in your neuroendocrine system and may cause either mood swings or depressive episodes.

A MISSING PIECE IN YOUR PUZZLE

Many people don't realize the extent to which the drugs they're using influence their body, so take a moment right now and jot down all the drugs you're presently using and any past drugs that you think might have adversely influenced you. Ask yourself if you've noticed any changes in your mood related to these drugs. Ask yourself if you remember any foods that have adversely influenced your mood. Read labels carefully and demand to know the possible side effects and interactions of all drugs that are prescribed for you.

The most important advice really is the one we give you in every chapter: Exclude PMS before you make any assumptions about the source of your problem. At least 40 percent of all women have some degree of PMS. If you have mood swings, there is a considerable likelihood that a shortage of brain fuel aggravated by Premenstrual Syndrome is behind it.

An Important Caution

In handling your problems with mood swings, depression, or any of the other potentially serious problems we discuss in this book, **it is essential not to discontinue your pre-scribed medications without discussing this first with your doctor!** The advice we give in this book is intended to make it possible for you to deal with your own premenstrual difficulties, but if you have other problems, or are already on serious medications, this book is not an effective substitute for the care by a qualified physician.

7

Anxiety and Tension

THIS CHAPTER WILL SHOW YOU:

- What anxiety and tension are
- How common anxiety and tension is in PMS sufferers
- How to tell if your anxiety and tension are PMS-related
- The caffeine connection
- How to lower your premenstrual irritability and tension

For a very long time—since the mid-1930s, in fact, which was perhaps even before your mothers heard of it—Premenstrual Syndrome was referred to as Premenstrual Tension. This was, of course, because tension and irritability are the most frequently observed characteristics of PMS. And if we add to these that state of apprehension that is usually called *anxiety*, then we can easily recognize the wide variety of problems that occur.

What Are Anxiety and Tension?

Anxiety is a fearful altering of perception—a sense of nameless dread. Anxiety can be acute, sudden in onset, and intense. It can last a short while or be chronic—less intense but longer in duration, lasting from days to months.

In anxiety, the fight-or-flight response is activated and many alarming physiological changes occur. These include increased heart rate, palpitations, stabbing chest pain, trembling, sweating, weakness, dizziness, nausea, feeling of unreality, sense of air hunger leading to hyperventilation, tingling or numbness at the extremities, fear of imminent death or catastrophe.

Chronic anxiety is associated with chronic fatigue, headaches, sleep disturbances, and many smooth muscle disruptions, for example in areas like the stomach and intestines.

Tension refers only to the physical manifestations of anxiety produced by the tensing and tightening of the skeletal muscles of the body. These include muscle pain, stiffness, tenderness, headache caused by tightened neck muscles, feelings of tightness in the throat, back pain, pain in extremities or joints.

Certainly well over 90 percent of our PMS patients experience some increase in anxiety and tension premenstrually.

A Family in Trouble

Jennifer C., a doting mother with three young children, was having a lot of trouble. She had incessant fights with her husband that were loud enough to make the neighbors close their windows and turn up the volume on their television sets. Her nerves were stretched like piano wires for almost half of every month; and she was constantly afraid during the premenstrual portion of her cycle that she would strike her children. Family life began to seem like a long series of embarrassments and debacles. One weekend the family even had to cancel their trip to Disneyland because of angry fights in the car.

Jennifer was treated for her irritability, and she and her husband, Bill, had some marriage counseling, which focused mostly on how little attention he paid to her. That was a real issue, but even after Bill got his act together and improved his behavior a bit, Jennifer's irritability persisted. The birth of their third child was followed by a postpartum depression, and for Jennifer and Bill it was all downhill from there. Their bad situation worsened over the next year and ended up in a separation.

Jennifer's life was in disarray. She was seeing a very competent therapist three times a week—imagine the cost—who was, however, rather slow to include PMS in his differential diagnosis. Eventually, the therapist saw the light, which was good for Jennifer, but the personal price she had paid for premenstrual tension and irritability was already a high one.

Once Again, It's Your Brain That's Taking a Beating!

Your tension and irritability is a sign that PMS is up to its usual tricks. Your brain is in brownout—it's struggling with a decreased fuel supply. This causes increased irritability of the neural tissue, and as a result, a tendency for the cerebrum to overreact to stimulation. This produces psychological symptoms, ranging from irritability to hypochondrical preoccupations, and it produces physical symptoms as well, such as muscular tension and a racing heart, tremors, sweating, even fatigue and sleep disturbances.

In fact, anxiety can dominate your day. It can take the form of free-floating, generalized foreboding, or it can appear more specifically as phobias, panic states, obsessions, or many other diverse and distressing responses.

For now let's simply say that tension and anxiety lead to life crises such as these:

- Fear, panic, fatigue
- Pain, headaches, sleep disturbances
- Fights with loved ones, colleagues, and friends
- Child abuse
- Career crises, job loss
- Separation and divorce

Since everyone wants to avoid troubles like this we suggest you take our simple Tension and Trouble Test.

Tension and Trouble Test

If PMS is behind your tension, anxiety, and irritability, you should be able to tell by answering these questions:

1. Are you experiencing feelings of fear, foreboding, dread, or terror premenstrually?

2. Do you find yourself avoiding situations or other people because you find yourself to anxious to cope with them?

3. Do you get into more conflicts with others premenstrually?

4. Do you do things impulsively out of anger, fear, or tension that you would not normally do?

5. List your most common irritable encounters:

At home: _____

With loved ones: _____

On the job: _____

Do they occur more often premenstrually? Answer *Yes* or *No* to each of the above.

6. Is your anxiety generalized, or does it take a special specific form, such as a phobic fear of going out? Any other special fears?

7. Do you suffer more from the physical signs of anxiety—heart racing, palpitations, sweating—premenstrually?

8. Are there any other ways you notice yourself getting anxious premenstrually? Make a list.

If you've answered "Yes" to one or more of the above, then you should take steps to deal with what is probably premenstrual tension and/or anxiety.

Caffeine: The Often Overlooked Culprit

Caffeine is bad news for your already compromised system. It can trigger your fight-or-flight response and send your irritability level racing up like a hurricane off the Gulf of Mexico. After all, caffeine is a potent drug.

Many people erroneously think caffeine means only coffee. Tea contains caffeine, too, and so do many soft drinks and many over-the-counter drugs.

Let's take a look at some of the undesirable effects of caffeine.

1. *It increases the body's production of prostaglandins.* Prostaglandins, a group of hormone-like substances whose levels are normally increased during the premenstrual period, have been strongly implicated as a cause of breast tenderness, arthritis, abdominal cramping, headaches, and backaches. In fact, it is known that aspirin and anti-arthritic drugs ameliorate the discomfort of dysmenorrhea by the inhibition of prostaglandin production.
2. *It functions as a diuretic.* Caffeine depletes the body of essential minerals—notably potassium and magnesium—and water-soluble vitamins. If these are already at a low level, the following symptoms develop: fatigue, depression, irritability, and migraines.
3. *It causes the release of adrenalin.* Caffeine *lowers* the blood sugar level in your body. Adrenalin is then released to raise this level, and can cause irritability, anxiety, tremors, panic, insomnia, fatigue, dizziness, lack of concentration, rage, and loss of memory.

We suggest that caffeine be cut down to a low level of intake or avoided altogether (not just during the premenstrual period). Cutting out caffeine only during the premenstrual period can cause withdrawal symptoms that are similar to PMS symptoms, aggravating them.

Hints to help you reduce your intake of caffeine:

- It is unhealthy to drink more than two cups of coffee a day. Start by reducing your intake by one cup a day.
- Read labels for hidden caffeine.
- Caffeine is found in, among other foods: coffees, teas, colas and other soft drinks, chocolate and over-the-counter medications such as stimulants (NoDoz®), aspirin compounds (Anacin®, Excedrin®, Midol®), and diet pills (Dexatrim®, for instance).
- Brew teas for less time.
- Use a coarser grind of coffee. The finer the grind, the higher the caffeine level content.
- Change the way you prepare coffee.
  The caffeine content in coffee varies depending on the method of preparation:

Blend and coffee brew	Amount of caffeine, per 5 oz. serving
Instant, decaffeinated	3 mg.
Instant, regular	66 mg.
Percolated	110 mg.
Drip method	146 mg.

- Substitute coffee with herbal teas (some have nutritional benefits), decaffeinated tea, decaffeinated coffee or coffee substitutes.
- When you drink coffee, be aware of: Where are you? What mood are you in? What friends are you with? What are you doing? It is important to know when you are most likely to drink coffee so that you can avoid the situation.
- Keep busy when the caffeine urge strikes. Try any of the following to help you overcome it: go for a walk, do relaxation exercises, exercise, and keep your hands busy.

Caffeine is a drug, a powerful stimulant, a member of the family of chemicals known as *xanthines*. Our best advice is for you not to take to much of it.

How to Lower Your Premenstrual Irritability and Tension

In the matter of tension and anxiety, you'll want to follow the same procedures you do for all other masks of PMS. Use your calendar. If the problem is a premenstrual one, your calendar will tell you. And if the problem is premenstrual, try to treat it by treating your PMS rather than by directly suppressing the symptoms.

In addition to the normal dietary changes that we advise, you can resolve *never to go more than three hours during your premenstruum without eating some of the recommended foods*. Following this rule will usually diminish your premenstrual irritability to a very manageable level—if you're on the right diet, and *if* you eliminate or at least minimize your caffeine intake.

Tranquilizers, for instance, are not a good idea if you can live life without them. Not only are they habituating, they can "fog you out" in your premenstrual period, further impairing your already somewhat impaired functioning. Doesn't it make a lot more sense to treat your PMS effectively, so you won't need to tranquilize yourself?

Anxiety disorders do exist. If after studying your menstrual calendar, you determine that your anxiety exists throughout the month or results from a specific traumatic experience, see a mental health professional.

8

Panic Attacks and Heart Problems

THIS CHAPTER WILL SHOW YOU:

- What panic attacks are
- Why women have more panic attacks than men
- How PMS-induced panic can get misdiagnosed as heart problems
- What the effects and dangers of current drug therapies for panic attacks are

Pam C. came in to see us because of her panic attacks. She was thirty-six, an active, cheerful woman and an avid, lifelong tennis player. But for the past three years she had been troubled by sudden, terrible panic attacks. She would feel paralyzing fear, break into a sweat, and become short of breath.

She had been to several doctors over a two-year period before our meeting with her. One of the doctors thought that her shortness of breath might be due to mitral valve prolapse. He heard a "click" through her thin chest wall. On his recommendation, she gave up tennis but the panic attacks persisted. Then she consulted other doctors. They couldn't pin down the heart problem, but they prescribed a variety of potent drugs for her panic. None of those drugs relieved her attacks for very long. Pam abandoned them, together with the physicians who had recommended them.

Then Pam noticed that her attacks invariably occurred in the week before her period, and that led her to us. Long story made short and clear: Pam took a stress test with cardiac monitoring; it was negative. We did a Glucose Tolerance Test which showed us a four-hour value of 44. Low blood sugar—as we suspected—which can increase the heart rate, was clearly indicated. We placed Pam on our nutritional treatment program.

End of panic attacks. Pam went back to playing tennis without any shortness of breath (except when she had to go back for three or four overhead lobs in a row).

What Are Panic Attacks?

The reality of panic attacks is pretty awful. We speak offhandedly of having "panicked" at discovering a wallet or a purse missing, and, in such a context, considerable anxiety is a natural reaction. When life-threatening danger appears, a more extreme response is normal. Adrenalin is quickly released, hormonally activating our fight-or-flight response. The heart rate accelerates and breathing quickens. We fight or we flee until the chemicals are spent and we return to normal.

But for sufferers of phobias, recurring panic attacks, or chronic anxiety, panic is not a momentary pulsation of fear; it is a paralyzing, life-limiting condition.

Panic attacks are sudden episodes of uncontrollable anxiety manifested by a pounding heart, weak, rubbery legs, chest pain, headache, dizziness, and trembling. There is frequently shortness of breath, flushing, tremors, and profuse sweating. The combination of intense fear and these physical reactions often causes the individual to believe he or she is going to die or is going crazy. There is often a compelling need to escape. Sufferers not only complain of sheer terror, but of a persistently heightened sense that everything might go wrong—what has been termed a "catastrophic overappraisal."

Some people experience an isolated panic attack only once or twice in a lifetime, but panic attacks become a disorder—often referred to as panic disorders—when these attacks of overwhelming anxiety occur with increasing frequency and magnitude over time.

CLINICAL CLUES

Do You Have Panic Attacks?

Do you have striking physical complaints such as racing heart beats (tachycardia), shortness of breath (dyspnea), dizziness, flushing, tremors, or profuse sweating?

Do you fear losing control, imminent death, or "going crazy?"

Do you have a fear of going out (agoraphobia), a desire to remain permanently in the safety of your home?

Do you get a heightened sense of dread that everything might go wrong in your life?

Do you have some degree of fatigue or depression (what a psychiatrist would call "secondary depression") added to your anxiety and/or panic? Does this depression lead to behavior like withdrawal from and phobic avoidance of situations that you perceive as threatening?

The most arresting and noteworthy statistic is that some studies have shown that *at least ten times as many women as men have such attacks*. Are women innately more panicky? We doubt it!

Then how does the medical profession attempt to account for this disproportion? Mostly by totally ignoring it! Until physicians with expertise in PMS began to appear, no one accounted for it or even seriously attempted to. And until most physicians include PMS in their differential diagnoses, panic attacks will remain a mystery.

Why Women Have a Lot of Panic Attacks

Those whose bias it is to think women the weaker sex naturally imagine that it's a sufficient explanation for the disproportionate occurrence of panic in women. But eons of recorded history—not to mention the insurance tables for life expectancy—clearly demonstrate that whatever women are, they're not the weaker sex. And the idea that women are subject to more panic doesn't really ring true either.

We believe the difference in the sex ratio can be due to only one thing: the inherent hormonal differences between men and women lead to drastically different propensities and symptoms. If you suffer from panic attacks, our experience indicates that it is most likely due to an abnormality in your blood sugar. More often than not that abnormality will turn out to be related to PMS. We know this because the great majority of panic attacks in women occur in the premenstrual period.

Although the timing of your panic attacks is the truest test of whether PMS is involved in their causation, let us just mention one very common pointer to where the trouble lies.

Have you ever had a panic attack wake you up in the night? Studies indicate that as many as 70 percent of patients with PMS report such an attack at least once. They wake up trembling in their sleep, filled with fear, and often bathed in perspiration.

But our clinic experience has repeatedly shown that *the most frequent cause of nighttime panic attacks is a drop in blood sugar*. The majority of middle-of-the-night panic attack sufferers have gone too long without eating. Their blood sugar drops too low, their hearts start racing, and they wake up in panic.

The simple remedy: Eat some type of complex carbohydrate combined with a small amount of protein right at bedtime. You might try a raw carrot and a small piece of cheese. Or a hardboiled egg and some lettuce and tomato.

If—as our clinical experience shows us—the vast majority of panic attacks are caused by PMS, then the mistreatment and misdiagnosis of panic attacks among women is epidemic and inexcusable. Let's see how that mistreatment unfolds in the case of one woman.

Panic on the Fast Track

Carla H., thirty-one, was a "fast-track" lady, the living proof that yuppies still exist—an Ivy league honors graduate of Harvard Business School—with a *big* job at a downtown Wall Street firm. Her life had been a roaring express train with one small stop for a two-year marriage. She was now single, with a nine-month-old daughter.

But postpartum (and post divorce), Carla began experiencing progressively disabling panic attacks. The crippling attacks were a real threat to her ability to work at the boardroom level. Being a no-hesitation, get-things-done kind of person, Carla looked for fast help. She saw a psychologist for two months. The experience was quite useful in dealing with the stress of her marital separation, but the panic attacks continued unabated. The psychologist began hinting that Carla was panicky because she had trouble accepting her maternal role after the birth of her daughter. Carla took one loving look at her daughter and walked out of that office permanently.

Next she went to a prominent psychiatrist, who put her on a tricyclic antidepressant named Tofranil®. It did nothing for her condition but constipated her and slowed down her thinking. The psychiatrist upped the dosage. That slowed down Carla's express train so much it almost stopped. Carla left him and tried relaxation therapy. It was a good therapy, but hardly effective against panic attacks. So Carla tried three more doctors and one of them finally put her on Xanax®.

Now here was a powerful therapy. The benzodiazepine, introduced by Upjohn in the early 1980s, is the only drug that the FDA has allowed to be advertised as specific for the panic attacks. At this very moment, Xanax® is being given to millions of women. It can be very effective, but unfortunately it can cause *severe* drowsiness, cognitive blurring, and addictive problems. It can also be such a difficult drug to stop that the intermediate use of yet another drug is required to ease withdrawal.

To her initial delight, Carla found that the Xanax® was working. She also found that she had to maintain blood levels of the medication that induced mental fogginess and physical drowsiness.

And then the Xanax® stopped working!

Carla had visions of her fast track career train finally derailing, and then she saw us mentioned in a book, and came to see us for treatment of you know what. Just one month on a proper diet demonstrated to Carla that her panic attacks were nothing more or less than a product of PMS. A little careful work with a calendar caused Carla to report that most of her attacks began at ovulation and got worse the closer she came to her period. We also found that she was drinking one glass of wine each evening—it was a sure-fire method of promoting PMS.

"But wine isn't really alcohol," Carla said.

"Oh no," we said, "and do you think also that soda doesn't have sugar?"

Carla promptly imposed the same no-nonsense approach to her nutritional treatment as she did to the rest of her life. She abandoned sugar and alcohol for half of every month, and she diligently ate the right sort of snack every three hours to keep her blood glucose level stable.

Is It Your Heart or Is It PMS?

Panic attacks have frequently merged with another headlined diagnosis of the 1980s—mitral valve prolapse. A diagnosis of MVP would imply that there is a difficulty with the mitral valve, one of the valves of the heart. Because it does not close properly, it disrupts the ability of the heart to pump effectively. The result is an accelerated rapid heart rate which often causes anxiety and panic attacks.

Mitral valve prolapse is by no means easy to diagnose accurately. Starting in the early 1980s, we saw a surge of women who were diagnosed as having mitral valve prolapse. Frequently these

Current Drug Therapy for Panic Attacks

Benzodiazepines. These are the most common form of treatment for anxiety attacks. Xanax® is the King of the Hill, having largely displaced the other popular benzodiazepines, Valium® (*diazepam*) and Ativan® (*lorazepam*) in this area. All of these drugs are quite effective initially, but they don't cure the disorder; their effectiveness usually wears off; they can be powerfully addictive; there is widespread overuse/abuse; and there is no evidence that they do more than mask the symptoms of a disorder whose underlying *cause* they never in any way address.

Tricyclic antidepressants (TCAs). TCAs have been shown to be effective in treating some forms of panic attacks. However, while initial reports indicated treatment effectiveness at relatively low doses (much lower than the doses that would be used in treating depression), some evidence has been forthcoming (and this is consistent with our own experience) that shows low doses to be ineffective. Higher doses are required, and this brings along such side effects as drowsiness, impaired concentration, constipation, postural hypotension, and sexual dysfunction.

Antihistamines. These anti-allergy drugs are actually prescribed for panic attacks because they have a sedative effect. They are not particularly effective and have side effects. And, again, they do nothing to address the underlying cause.

Alcohol. Alcohol is mostly a self-administered solution to panic, though some doctors will say, "If you feel that way, why don't you have a glass of wine." Of course, the side effects and addictive properties of alcohol are too well known to need discussion here. Its long-term effectiveness against panic is not great, and if you have PMS panic, alcohol will worsen it.

Buspirone. This newer, very mild anti-anxiety medication has been used extensively because it has little potential for addiction. However, it is generally a very weak tranquilizer.

Barbituates. These old-fashioned sleep medications are potentially dangerous, addictive, and should not be used for panic attacks.

Phenothiazines. Using these very strong drugs (Haldol®, Thorazine®, Stelazine®, Mellaril®, among others) is clearly overkill. They don't treat panic, except by absolutely immobilizing the patient, and they have absolutely hideous side effects when used longterm. Phenothiazines are so potentially dangerous that they should be used only for psychosis and other similarly severe disorders. They are inappropriate for panic attacks and anxiety-related neuroses.

MAO Inhibitors. These drugs (Nardil®, Parnate®, etc.) are another form of antidepressant that sometimes work in cases where the patient doesn't respond to other medication. However, they represent an *absolutely* last line of treatment and are far more dangerous than any of the other drugs we mentioned.

were athletic women with thin chest walls that led to louder heart sounds when a doctor listened to their heart sounds with a stethoscope.

Pam C., whose story opened this chapter, was an excellent and rather standard example of mitral valve misdiagnosis. A girl who provided a more unusual example of the confusion of panic attacks with heart disorders came in for a visit recently. Patricia C., fourteen years old, arrived in our office on St. Patrick's Day wearing a radiant smile and a sweatshirt saying "Irish Princess." Her vibrancy illuminated the far corners of the waiting room, even though this Irish Princess had devastating panic attacks that were impairing her life and limiting her exuberant teenage behavior. Moreover, she had a major medical history behind her, having been operated on as a young infant for transposition of her major heart vessels—a problem that still caused her to lose her breath frequently.

Her cardiologists believed her panic attacks were due to her heart problem. Her perceptive mother, a social worker, noted that they only occurred premenstrually. Perhaps what nailed down the conclusion for her was the fact that her older daughter also had panic attacks premenstrually.

We assumed that changing her nutrition within the parameters explained in this book would enable her to function at a more normal level of life. We knew we would have to work closely with her cardiologists, and we did so. Once the diagnosis of PMS was clear, and the panic attacks began to abate, they were perfectly willing to accept the conclusion that this was not an aspect of her heart problem.

What Has the Medical World Been Doing?

The medical world has been treating panic attacks with standard pharmaceutical protocols and having some success with some of the people whose condition is not induced by PMS. Imipramine® and other antidepressants have been widely prescribed and often result in improvements.

As for Xanax®, its impact has been so great that the American Psychiatric Association promoted panic attacks to the status of a major entity in its standard diagnostic manual, the *DSM III*. Unfortunately, Xanax® will do you little good if your real problem is PMS.

What You Can Do Right Now

First, keep charting.

If your panic attacks are more prevalent premenstrually, make sure you get an accurate Glucose Tolerance Test immediately before menstruation—while you have symptoms. Follow the nutritional treatment program (see chapter 15) diligently and be particularly careful to eat six small meals a day including something just before bedtime so your blood sugar won't drop during your sleep.

This has proven to be especially effective in relieving PMS-related panic attacks and other anxiety symptoms.

9

Headaches

THIS CHAPTER WILL SHOW YOU:

- The various types of headaches
- What causes headaches
- How to tell if your headaches are PMS-related
- How hormones and headaches are related
- How hypoglycemia can cause your headache
- How to use a Food Journal and a Stress Journal to eliminate your headache triggers
- How you can treat a PMS headache

Headaches, particularly migraines, are one of the most frequent complaints of the women we see with PMS. Over 50 percent of our patients complain of severe, recurring headaches that have not been alleviated by treatment. According to the National Headache Institute, an estimated 18 million people in the United States suffer from migraine headaches, and 79 percent of them are women. Such headaches cause sufferers to miss an average of nine days from work each year at a cost of $50 billion to their employers.

Not all the headaches that women get are caused by PMS, but a substantial percentage of them are, and, as you might imagine, a huge proportion of those are misdiagnosed and mistreated.

If you suffer from headaches, and you follow this chapter carefully, you will find a complete system for determining the cause of your headaches and establishing their relationship to your menstrual cycle. If they are related to your PMS, you will be able to start treating them immediately.

Your headaches should never receive extensive treatment without your first taking a pencil and a calendar and figuring out to what extent they occur in the premenstruum.

Tension Headaches

The most common form of headache is a tension headache. This is often assumed to be caused by tightening of the muscles in the back of the neck. But it may also be a form of vascular headache, similar in that respect (though not in other respects) to the mechanism for migraine headache. The tension headache is usually caused by stress and very often is set in motion by going too long without eating. Chronic anxiety, since it causes changes in muscle tension, can also trigger tension headache.

Migraines

The migraine is a type of headache caused by dilation (swelling) of the blood vessels located under your skull and on the outside of your brain. It is usually the severest form of vascular headache. The problem in all vascular headaches is that the outer lining of our heads has an incredibly dense concentration of blood vessels; when those blood vessels swell or dilate, they press upon the nerves in the head and produce pain. Migraines are divided into two types, *classical* and *common*. Both are marked by pain (frequently severe or incapacitating) on one or both sides of the head, by intolerance to light or noise, and may be accompanied by nausea or vomiting.

In the *classical* variety of migraine, a warning, called an aura, comes before the onset of a severe headache. These auras may take the form of patterns of light, brightly colored stars or stripes, or a patch of blindness in one area of your visual field. Other sensory changes include feelings of excitability, altered muscle tone, tics, and even variations in memory and speech. The *common* migraine does not have an aura and begins gradually, increasing in severity.

Both forms of migraine can last anywhere from several hours to several days.

The definitions and names for headaches are legion, sometimes overlapping, and frequently controversial as far as the headache experts are concerned. Let's just say that there are many other types of headaches such as sinus headaches, histamine headaches, and cluster headaches (regarded by many as a form of migraine.)

Causes Galore

In our experience, the most common environmental factor triggering a PMS headache is skipping a meal or allowing too long a time to pass between one meal and the next. This is, of course, related to the lowering of blood sugar levels, and we'll say a little more about it a little further on in the chapter.

Headaches also commonly result when the headache sufferer has a sensitivity to certain foods. There are virtually no foods to which someone is not intolerant, but fortunately most sufferers are affected by similar foods. High on the list are chocolate, citrus fruits, aged cheese, pork, meats such as sausage and hot dogs that contain sodium nitrate, and alcohol. Champagne and red wine are particularly potent provokers of headaches, especially migraines. Foods (particularly Chinese restaurant food) containing the meat tenderizer and flavor enhancer monosodium glutamate (MSG) have been frequently linked to migraine attacks.

Another frequent trigger is exposure to bright sunlight. Some specialists say the incidence of headaches rises in the summer when people garden or exercise on sunny days, sit outside for picnics and baseball games, or merely drive along the highway into a bright glare.

Some patients also report suffering from headaches after a day on the ski slopes when the paler winter sun reflects off the snow. There's also evidence that the phosphorescent glow of a computer screen can provoke an attack of migraine or other headache.

Are Your Headaches PMS-Related?

The hormonal changes in a woman's body during the premen-struum frequently set the stage for a headache. There is some theoretical understanding of how and why this occurs. What we normally find is that a woman with a tendency to suffer from headaches will be affected by certain physical changes occurring in the premenstrual period and thus may end up with an unusually large number of headaches as part of her PMS pattern. But before we can discuss the causes and the treatment of headaches that occur premenstrually, you should take a calendar and a pencil and attempt to answer the obvious questions:

1. Do your headaches occur premenstrually?
2. Do they occur at other times of the month but become more frequent or more severe premenstrually?
3. Do they occur randomly, with no apparent relation to your menstrual cycle?

If you answered "yes" to question No. 3, PMS is unlikely to play a role in your headaches, but a "yes" to the first two questions means that PMS is almost certainly implicated in the causation of your headaches.

In 1975, a study of 886 women who suffered from migraine attacks by the British Migraine Association showed that there were clearly two groups: those whose attacks appeared to be hormon-ally related and those whose migraines were sporadic. The women whose headaches appeared to be related to their menstrual cycle showed many of the following characteristics. We suggest you test yourself further.

- Did your headaches have their onset at puberty, or after first taking contraceptive pills, or after a pregnancy?
- Did the attacks occur at approximately the same time in each menstrual cycle?
- Were you free from attacks in the later stages of pregnancy?

- Was there an increase in the severity of your headaches after each pregnancy (or each abortion or miscarriage)?

What If You Don't Look for PMS?

It's possible to suffer headache pain for a long time without ever closing in on a real solution.

Donna M., forty-three, a mother and housewife, was a very typical patient of ours. She had had migraines for *more than twenty years*. The pain was frequently devastating, and it would lay her flat in a darkened room for hours on end. Naturally, she sought help. Her family doctor prescribed a series of painkillers for her—Fiorinal®, Percocet®—and then noticed, a little bit late, that they were leading her toward addiction.

Donna's doctor then tried to wean her off the painkillers with tranquilizers, but it wasn't easy. Besides, all the medication she was taking was making her so sleepy that she could barely function. Finally, after she had a minor auto accident while driving the kids to school, everyone made a serious effort to get her off the medications. But the headaches still continued to distress her.

Donna went to a headache clinic and saw an eminent specialist in the field. He did a long series of diagnostic tests culminating in an expensive CAT scan and an MRI. While all these tests were being done, he was trying her out on Inderal® and Elavil®. Inderal® blocks peripheral nerve receptor sites and is sometimes used to

---

CLINICAL CLUES

Are your headaches limited to one spot in your head or do they move about? If they are limited to one area, they are more likely due to a specific underlying cause such as sinuses, infected teeth, or nerve damage. PMS headaches, in general, tend to be vague or migratory in location.

prevent the onset of migraines; Elavil® is an antidepressant, which has a side effect of toning down your nervous system. The Inderal® worked for a while, but the migraines came back with increased severity.

Meanwhile, Donna had a terrifying night waiting for the CAT scan and MRI to image the inside of her head. The specialist had indicated some of the things he was trying to rule out with these highly sophisticated and enormously expensive tests, and they had included multiple sclerosis and a brain tumor.

"What will I tell my children if I'm dying of a brain tumor?" Donna found herself wondering.

She didn't realize that her specialist didn't for a moment believe that she had either of these problems. He saw thousands of patients with pain in their heads, and these tests were, for him, simply standard. They seldom revealed anything significant, but when they did, he felt justified in having ordered them. Besides, if he didn't order them, he could be sued for malpractice.

Happily, Donna's results arrived almost immediately and were completely negative. An expensive medical workup so far, but Donna still had her headaches.

Donna's next step was a fortunate one. On the recommendation of a friend, she came to our center, and we soon saw that PMS was a major component in her migraines.

Before we tell you more about Donna, we'll explain what it is about the changes in a woman's body in the premenstrual period that can result in headaches.

Headaches and PMS

There are at least two main mechanisms by which PMS causes headaches.

As we've already seen, estrogen and progesterone, the two main female hormones, both increase markedly at the time of ovulation. The increase in estrogen alone may, in fact, be one of the causes of headache. Since estrogen binds salt in the body and salt binds water, high levels of the hormone may lead to edema, or fluid retention. Such edema may not only cause the swelling of stomach, breasts, and legs that can be such an uncomfortable aspect of the premenstrual period, it may also cause a swelling of tissue in the brain. However, the brain can only expand a very small amount because the skull is rigid. Since the bed of nerves that lies between the skull and the brain is very sensitive to pressure, one of the results is pain. This pressure can also lead to a wide range of other symptoms, including the inability to concentrate, dizziness, and, in rare instances, seizures. But for the purpose of this chapter, the symptom we'll deal with is pain.

Hypoglycemia is also relevant. It has been demonstrated that as little as a 5 percent drop in blood sugar can cause symptoms of nerve deprivation in the brain. Once the supply of glucose to the brain begins to drop because the percentage of glucose in the blood is lower than normal, the body adapts by increasing the volume of blood flowing to the brain. This is a sure-fire formula for creating a vascular headache if you have even the slightest tendency to headaches. But this situation can usually be prevented if you follow the recommendations for avoiding premenstrual hypoglycemia. Going too long without eating and eating the wrong foods at the wrong time of the month are guaranteed to bring on a hypoglycemic headache.

In addition to these two absolutely clear methods of creating headache, there is the always vexing question of stress. Some doctors feel that stress alone can bring on headaches, and certainly for women with PMS that whole portion of the month is stressful. It's possible, however, that it's not so much stress as it is the things that stress makes one do that leads to a pain in the head. In any event, stress has to be taken seriously, and it's something you certainly need to control in your life.

A Happy Outcome for Donna

Now let's go back to Donna M. Tracing the connection between headache and PMS requires precise calendar work—we call it a *Three Pencil Problem*. Donna was more than happy to oblige. We discovered that although Donna had headaches throughout the premenstrual period, they *peaked at ovulation*, the moment when estrogen spikes upward. We suspected that her headaches were hormonal and hypoglycemic in origin.

First, we put her on our nutritional program to help control her low blood sugar. This was successful as far as it went. The headaches decreased and on Donna's self-rating scale she had improved 40 percent.

We still had her hormonal problem to deal with, so we added natural progesterone—300 mgs. of the oral micronized tablets twice a day during her premenstrual phase. Experience has shown that extra progesterone can control the effects of high estrogen levels at that time of the month.

This treatment was almost a complete success. Donna's headaches diminished by approximately 95 percent. After so many years of suffering, she regarded this as next of kin to a miracle.

Then we had a temporary setback. Two months after the big breakthrough, Donna's headaches returned. Clearly there was something we were missing. We had asked Donna to keep a Stress Journal and a Food Journal when we first started working with her. It took only a brief look at these records to discover the causes of Donna's setback.

CLINICAL CLUE

Avoid Precipitating Foods!

The most frequent trigger of headaches is going too long without eating. But you must also look carefully at what you eat.

Migraines may be triggered by the body's sensitivity to certain food. The attack may occur not when the food is being digested by the stomach, but twelve to thirty-six hours later, when it is broken down by the liver. The breakdown products are substances (vasodilating amines) that

---

are capable of dilating the blood vessels of the brain, thereby allowing an excessive surge of blood into the head. This is felt as throbbing pain.

The two most common vasodilating amines are tyramine (found in aged cheeses), and phenylethylamine (found in alcohol and chocolate). During the premenstrual phase, a woman prone to migraines is sensitive not only to the above foods but also to the other foods listed below.

Foods to Avoid

- *Tyramine* is not present in cream or cottage cheese, only in mature or aged cheeses. Particular cheeses to avoid are: Stilton and other blue cheeses, Cheddar, Parmesan, and processed cheeses. Warning: Mature cheese is hidden in quiches, Mornay sauce, and many Italian dishes.
- *Alcohols* found to provoke migraines are: red wine, sherry, port, and champagne. (In addition, alcohol contains sugar which causes hypoglycemic dysfunction.) More people are sensitive to grape alcohols than to grain alcohols like beer and whiskey.
- *Chocolate* should be avoided entirely. Be careful for hidden chocolate (added for color) in rich fruit cakes, ginger cakes, coffee dishes, and many other party dishes. Chocolate cravings can indicate a magnesium deficiency.
- *Citrus fruits* should be avoided. Don't forget that this also includes mandarins and tangerines, along with oranges, lemons, grapes, and grapefruits.
- *Other foods* to which there may be an increased sensitivity: pork, onions, ripe bananas, fish.

A Food Journal—Lag Times

If you have recurring migraines, it is essential that you keep a careful and accurate record of exactly what you eat and drink. Record the times of the day you do it, what quantities you ingest, and exactly what the food and drink is. It's very possible that if you remove some of the foods we mentioned earlier in the chapter, your headaches may die down or disappear altogether. It's also possible that you may find there are other foods that you can associate with the onset of headaches. Naturally, in keeping a food journal for this purpose, you should also keep a record of the days and times of your headaches.

Pay attention to the lag—the interval between eating a certain food and the onset of a headache. You may be able to notice characteristic lag times between the ingestion of certain foods and the start of your pain.

Your Stress Journal

You can easily keep track of stress as part of your Food Journal (see page 160 for an example) by the use of asterisks. Just put one asterisk, or two, or three next to the time when some slightly, or significantly, or tremendously stressful event occurs in your life.

You might have a fight with your boyfriend about what time to meet for a movie—that might be a one-asterisk event (or two, depending on the state of the relationship). On the other hand, if someone you love has a heart attack, that will probably be a three-asterisk event, assuming you have the strength and will to record it.

If *stress* is one of the factors in your headaches, you'll soon begin to see a relationship to those asterisks and the onset of headache pain.

Donna's journal was filled with asterisks. Her husband had left one job and was looking for another. Her mother was in the hospital. The result of all that stress showed up in her Food Journal. Donna had reverted to drinking an occasional glass of red wine. It took just a minute to trace the connection between the stress, the alcohol and the headaches. Just another example of how essential good record-keeping is when it comes to handling your PMS.

Unmasking the Source of Your Headache

Let's take a quick look at some of the questions you ought to be asking yourself if you're a woman with headaches.

1. Do your headaches occur only premenstrually?
2. Do they occur at other times of the month but more frequently premenstrually?
3. Are they related to alcohol, to the consumption of any particular foods, or to going too long without eating? (Note that alcohol can cause headaches up to 36 hours later!)
4. Does stress bring them on?
5. Does stress make them worse?
6. Do they occur at certain times of the day?
7. Does getting up suddenly from a sitting position make them worse? That could be due to a sudden drop in blood pressure called postural hypotension.
8. Are you on any medication that might be causing the headaches? Certain medications like Sudafed® can raise blood pressure and cause headaches.
9. Does anything relieve the headaches significantly?
10. What foods, if any, make it worse?
11. Do you have allergies?
12. Do you have recurrent sinusitis?
13. Do you have vaginal yeast infections? Have you ever had them in other parts of the body? (For more information on yeast infections, see chapter 21.)
14. Have you had your blood pressure checked? What is it? You need to know. Headaches on awakening may be due to a high blood pressure.

CLINICAL CLUE

The Test Dose

For those difficult-to-handle premenstrual headaches, a test dose of natural progesterone can be the solution. It generally works best on headaches that occur at highly specific days of the month.

You need your doctor to prescribe a single dose of oral progesterone. He should understand the dosage. A dose of only 50 mgs. will be ineffective; 200 or 300 mgs. of the oral micronized form are necessary to get results. You must take the progesterone before your headache really gets started. Once the headache is well under way, the progesterone will be ineffective.

Two very important points:
1. Make sure you get natural progesterone.
2. Take it early enough and in sufficient quantities.

In summary, our experience has been that there are few more common masks for PMS than headache. If you can track your headaches to your premenstrual period, you will surely be able to lessen them.

10

Alcoholism

THIS CHAPTER WILL SHOW YOU:

- The difference between alcohol intolerance and episodic alcoholism
- The damage that alcohol can do to women
- Why that damage is intensified premenstrually
- The connection between alcohol and low blood sugar
- How to tell if you have a drinking problem

It would be hard to overstate the effect alcohol has on premenstrual women.

Take Cassie, who called us and in a soft voice, asked for a "private consultation." Arriving breathless a few minutes late for her appointment, she looked stunning in a powder blue workout outfit, her lovely blonde hair fashionably drawn back under a headband. Sweating slightly, she was still a strikingly beautiful woman, pleasant and softspoken. We weren't surprised to learn she had once been an actress.

Her story wasn't as beautiful. She was married to an aging American statesman. It was her third marriage and it was beginning to go terribly wrong.

Each and every month, she and her husband would have terrible arguments. She would start drinking; one glass of scotch would follow another, and then the argument would escalate to the shouting stage. Very often it would then progress to violence—Cassie would stalk her husband through their Park Avenue duplex and begin assaulting him.

CLINICAL CLUE

If you are asking yourself if you have a drinking problem, then you do! In all our years of seeing patients, we have never seen anyone who came in saying, "I'm not sure if I have a drinking problem," who turned out *not* to have a problem with alcohol.

If you are asking the question, you have the problem, and if you're a woman with PMS, then you only need to ask yourself how you are going to stop drinking—Period! (Sorry to be so hard-line, but you can't afford to waste any more of your life.) There's no such thing as being able to drink a little if you have PMS-alcohol-intolerance.

It was hard to imagine this softspoken, gracious, and beautiful woman beating anyone up. But she assured me it was all quite true. It had started some four years ago, in her late thirties, following a tubal ligation after the birth of her third child.

Since then she had PMS, and her premenstrual problem had intensified with alcohol. In the week before her period, she would find herself drinking incessantly and then things would spiral downhill. Ironically, she was very fond of her husband, and he was very fond of her, and they had a great relationship the rest of the month.

He came in the next day, thirty minutes late because he had to wait for a telephone call from the President! A very polite, distinguished gentleman but a little too busy and clouded with his own self-importance to listen carefully to what was wrong with his wife.

As for Cassie the story never did get right. She led too self-indulgent a life style to give up drinking entirely for half of each month.

Except for the exalted social status of the people involved, *there was nothing unusual* about this story.

Women and Alcohol

There are many critical misconceptions about drinking and the American woman.

- Six out of ten American women drink.
- Of those who drink, 95 percent are light drinkers (three drinks a week) to moderate drinkers (one drink a day).
- Women tend to take a drink to "relax," while men drink to be "more sociable."
- Women who are more likely to drink include: women with college degrees, women with annual household incomes over $50,000, women with strong religious ties.
- Women with multiple roles and responsibilities are reported to have fewer problems with alcohol than women with fewer life demands.
- Women alcoholics tend to die earlier not only from liver disease but from suicide, accidents, and circulatory disorders.

There probably is some correlation—though it hasn't yet been studied—between the *hypoglycemic depression* induced by PMS and the *extremely heavy rate of suicide attempts recorded premenstrually*—and this may also be related to the fact that women drink more premenstrually, and tend to combine drinking with sedatives and/or antidepressants, which is potentially a lethal combination. *And, as you know, misdiagnosis of PMS often leads to mistreatment characterized by the prescribing of those very same sedatives and antidepressants.*

Men and Women and Alcohol: Unequal Metabolisms

There are an estimated fifteen million alcohol abusers in the United States and approximately four million of them are women.

A Math Problem in Alcohol— A Myth Problem About Wine

Wine is seriously underestimated as a source of alcohol and a risk for alcohol-related problems.

Consider the following fact: Alcohol is alcohol. How much you get when you drink has to do with concentration and volume.

The amount of alcohol in—

- a glass of wine (5 oz. at 12% alcohol);
- a mug of beer (12 oz. at 5% alcohol); and
- a shot of hard liquor (1½ oz at 40% alcohol—80 proof)

is *almost exactly the same*. The percent of alcohol is adjusted for volume: The lower percentage of alcohol in beer or wine simply means you get a bigger glass.

Mostly, they're between the ages of thirty-five and forty-nine. Considering that they make up less than a third of the total number of alcohol abusers, women suffer a tremendously disproportionate number of health problems as a result of heavy drinking. (Note: thirty-five to forty-nine is when PMS is most common and severe.)

According to experts at John Hopkins Medical School, women arrive at a state of complete dependence on alcohol three or four times faster than men, and descend into the depths of the alcoholic abyss within five years of commencing heavy drinking, as opposed to fifteen to twenty years for men.

Physically, women are far less well equipped to handle alcohol than men. This is one area in which there isn't a shred of equality between the sexes!

Women, on average, are smaller and weigh less than men. The same quantity of alcohol will intoxicate them faster. Pound for pound women have more fatty tissue and men more muscle. Fat contains less water than muscle, so alcohol remains concentrated in a woman's body for a significantly longer time than in a man's simply because there's less water to dilute it.

In the event that a particular woman was as large as a particular man and was unusually fit and muscular, while he was unusually fat and flabby, she would still be remarkably disadvantaged. A man's stomach contains four times as much of the enzyme alcohol dehydrogenase as a woman's does, and the body uses that enzyme to metabolize and detoxify alcohol. Hence far more alcohol will reach a woman's liver, brain, and other organs. In addition, there is evidence that the female hormone estrogen combines with alcohol to exacerbate liver damage. Consequently, among the heaviest drinkers, women develop cirrhosis and hepatitis after a shorter period and at a lower level of daily drinking than men.

Alcohol and Low Blood Sugar

It is a well-established fact that women with PMS have a markedly diminished tolerance for alcohol. In fact, female alcoholics almost invariably state that their alcoholism is intensified during the premenstrual period and many of them add that their drinking problems started during their premenstrual days.

Alcohol brings about a startling intensification of many of the symptoms of PMS. By now you realize what a major role hypoglycemia plays in Premenstrual Syndrome. Well, *alcohol is a sugar: potentially the most dangerous form of glucose available.* It causes an overly rapid rise in blood sugar. This is followed by a tremendously over-reactive release of insulin, driving the blood sugar to dangerously low levels for extended periods. Since low blood sugar is responsible for much of the anger, irritability, and depression of PMS, you must face what alcohol can do to you.

Alcohol has a markedly worse effect than other sugars because, in an explosive secondary reaction, *it inhibits gluconeogenesis* (the process in which your metabolism breaks down reserves of glycogen—a storage form of glucose—to create more glucose when your blood sugar is low).

But, if you have even minute quantities of alcohol in your system, this metabolic response can be so disrupted that your hypoglycemia will last for two or three days. Thus the effects of a good wine at dinner may be felt not merely that night but for the next couple of days.

The relationship between alcohol and hypoglycemia has become so well known that many alcohol treatment centers have taken to recommending a modified hypoglycemic diet. One of our closest medical associates, Dr. Nicholas Pace, a renowned alcoholism specialist, carefully treats female alcoholics with a complete nutritional approach including vitamins and minerals. Over the years, he has taken to supplementing his program with Glucose Tolerance Tests when indicated.

Remember that hypoglycemia is not only the result of drinking but also a promoter of drinking. After all, a woman with a drinking problem will generally deal with the need for a sugar fix caused by a low level of blood sugar in the way she knows best—she'll have a drink. Thus the two conditions are closely intertwined.

CLINICAL CLUE

Do you crave sweets premenstrually? If alcohol is a problem for you during the premenstruum, there is certainly a direct connection. The craving for alcohol is, in fact, your body's way of attempting to replenish the supply of glucose in our blood. Alcohol shoots sugar into your bloodstream as rapidly as any substance because it is absorbed in the stomach. Unfortunately, it also causes your insulin to overreact more strongly than most other substances, thus bringing about a renewed state of lowered blood sugar and a desire for still more alcohol.

Can You Give Up Alcohol During the Premenstruum—Or Even All Month Long?

Some women experience strong resistance even on this issue.

Jeanne Marie was one of these. Alcohol had seemed to play a very minor part in her life. She was in her forties, lived in a country-club suburb and thoroughly enjoyed the "good life." She had a loving husband and two grown children who were well aware that there would be a couple of days each month when mom would be impossible to live with and dangerous to speak to. Her husband even had a standing arrangement with a local motel to sleep over for a night or two when things got really bad.

Jeanne Marie came to our center because of this extreme premenstrual irritability, as well as some very distressing breast tenderness.

On our standard health history form, there is a question which simply says, "Do you drink?" The answer we received was "No."

Somewhere in the course of the subsequent interview, we asked, "You don't drink alcohol at all?"

"No, no hard alcohol."

"Hard alcohol?"

"Yes, I only drink wine."

"But wine is alcohol."

"But it's not *hard* alcohol."

At this point we sighed and asked her how often she drank.

"Only when we go out to dinner [which for Jeanne Marie was four to seven times a week] . . . and besides, I never drink. I only have wine."

Next came a very leading question when it comes to alcohol and PMS. "Does alcohol affect you more premenstrually?"

"I never noticed."

"Well, tell me, Jeanne Marie, if you drink wine premenstrually do you get these angry outbursts the next day?"

Jeanne Marie gave me a hard, white stare and said, "Are you trying to tell me that I can't drink wine with my meals?"

Do You Have a Drinking Problem?

If you think you might, take this simple test.

1. Do you drink more than one drink a day?
2. Do you have any memory lapses after drinking?
3. Do you tend to gulp your drinks?
4. Once you start, are you unable to stop drinking until intoxicated?
5. Do you find that you will drink if there is alcohol in the house?
6. Are you ever tempted to take a drink before noon?
7. Do you think during the day about how great that drink will make you feel?
8. Do you open a bottle of wine to have one glass only to realize later that you've had two-thirds of the bottle?

Unbelievably, If you answered "yes" to any one of these questions, you probably are experiencing difficulties with the effects of alcohol.

As you can readily imagine from this dialogue, we did not have an easy time of it.

It is so difficult to communicate that the glowing candlelight dinner, the romantic restaurant, the elegant food accompanied by the silky Chardonnay, or the full-flavored Beaune, adds up to something not to be desired during the premenstrual days. What follows the day after is the crashing irritability and the crushing depression. And those are after-effects that may continue for days.

What has been clear to us, in our years of working with women's menstrual problems, is that alcohol is one of the worst possible aggravators of PMS and that PMS will certainly aggravate any pre-existing alcohol problems.

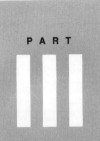

OTHER CONDITIONS RELATED TO THE HORMONAL CYCLE

11

Dysmenorrhea

THIS CHAPTER WILL SHOW YOU:

- The different types of dysmenorrhea
- Other sources of pelvic pain
- How menstrual pain is treated

Dysmenorrhea (menstrual pain) is not necessarily PMS, but it is often related to it, and we think it is important for you to know about the different common types.

Spasmodic Dysmenorrhea

Spasmodic dysmenorrhea is a hormonal and structural disorder of younger women. It usually begins between the ages of fifteen and twenty-five. It appears to be caused by an insufficient supply of estrogen for the proper development and stretching of the muscles of the uterus. Pregnancy to term will end this problem, since large amounts of estrogen are produced by the placenta, and the uterus is stretched by the fetus.

Doctors commonly treat spasmodic dysmenorrhea with either antiprostaglandins (like Motrin®, Advil®, Ponstel®) or with oral contraceptives. As you know, we would recommend that women avoid oral contraceptives whenever possible, and therefore, anti-prostaglandins are our medication of choice.

Prostaglandins are hormonelike substances that are usually present in higher levels in your uterus but are also found in a number of body tissues. Women who have painful menstrual

---

Do You Have Spasmodic Dysmenorrhea?

Some of the questions you should ask yourself are the following:

1. Does the pain usually start on the first day of your period?

2. Is the pain cramp-like (intermittent, piercing, and sharp), and is it usually limited to the lower abdomen, the back, and the external genital areas?

3. Did it stop after your first pregnancy? In the absence of pregnancy, is it diminishing as you grow older?

4. Is it relieved by the use of oral contraceptives?

If "yes" you probably have some form of dysmenorrhea. This pain is *not* PMS. Although, it is related to your menstrual cycle, it is not premenstrual.

---

cramps have been found to have more prostaglandins than women who do not.

In spasmodic dysmenorrhea, high levels of F-2 alpha, a particular prostaglandin, are secreted by the cells of the uterus. This is where antiprostaglandins come in. The commonest ones, such as Advil® and Motrin® (*ibuprofen*), are very familiar and can now be purchased over the counter. Some other common ones include Ponstel® (*mefenamic acid*), and Anaprox® (*sodium naproxen*). These drugs are being developed rapidly; new ones are entering the market every year. If you have to take one, take it with some food such as a cracker to avoid gastric distress.

In our practice, we seldom see pure cases of spasmodic dysmenorrhea. This condition is generally treated by the family doctor or gynecologist. In some cases of extreme pain, the gynecologist may even recommend a D & C to stretch the uterine opening.

Congestive Dysmenorrhea

Congestive dysmenorrhea is more closely associated with Premenstrual Syndrome. It is related to fluid retention and shows the following characteristics.

1. It may begin as many as four days before menstruation and then peak at first or second day of menstrual flow.
2. It can occur at any age. Women from fifteen to fifty-five can be affected.
3. The pain is usually not as sharp as the pain of spasmodic dysmenorrhea, but is more diffuse and is accompanied by lingering fatigue and a general sense of physical heaviness. The pain can occur in the lower abdomen, back, head, breast, joints, and limbs.
4. The use of the oral contraceptive pill increases fluid retention, and can increase the pain. (In spasmodic dysmenorrhea, on the other hand, the pain is relieved by the Pill.)
5. Pregnancy and aging may increase the symptoms.
6. It can usually be treated effectively with proper nutrition. Natural progesterone, which has a diuretic effect, can also be an effective treatment.

Endometriosis

Endometriosis is a less frequent form of cyclic pain related to the displacement of endometrial cells. (The endometrium is the lining of the uterus.) These cells can travel through the body and end up in the muscle wall or on the outside of the uterus or on the pelvic ligaments.

The endometrial cells react to hormonal changes at menstruation; they multiply or decrease in number in relation to your menstrual cycle. In this type of disorder, it is essential to have a good working relationship with your gynecologist; the treatment of endometriosis can be complicated. The good news is that the emergence of relatively sophisticated techniques of laporoscopy and laser surgery has made great inroads in the treatment of this insidious, painful, and often difficult-to-handle disorder.

In many cases of endometriosis, there is even better news. We have seen well over 60 percent of our patients improve greatly simply by following our PMS program. The elimination of fluid-retaining substances from the diet, coupled, when necessary, with natural progesterone, which opposes the fluid-retaining effects of estrogen, provides great relief for a number of patients.

Some Other Sources of Pelvic Pain

Pain, particularly pelvic pain, is not always easy to diagnose. There are other important causes of pain which might be confused with pain related to your menstrual cycle.

Ovarian cysts can cause a sharp, debilitating pain that is often difficult to diagnose because the cysts decrease in size or even "disappear" at times. For this reason, it's important to be examined while you're having this type of pain so that your gynecologist will be better able to make a correct diagnosis. Sonograms and laporoscopy help to diagnose this ailment.

Fibroids or other tumors can also cause pain. It is essential that, if you have continued pain in your lower abdomen (the pelvic area), that you maintain an ongoing relationship with your gynecologist until the pain is either ameliorated or eliminated. It simply isn't wise to leave pain undiagnosed or untreated. It is also possible for pelvic pain to be rather trickily "referred" from other parts of your body, such as your appendix. In such a case, you would feel pelvic pain although the medical problem would actually exist in another part of your body.

Dealing With Your Menstrual Pain

There is a wide variety of menstrual pain. You'll have to deal with it, certainly, but you don't have to accept it passively. With proper care and well-informed medical attention, most pain due to dysmenorrhea can be controlled. Sometimes it can be reduced to a very manageable or even insignificant level. As we've seen, dietary changes alone will satisfactorily alleviate the suffering in certain cases. If you can do it, you will certainly find that that's a far better solution than dependence on drugs.

12

Postpartum Depression

THIS CHAPTER WILL SHOW YOU:

- What causes postpartum depression
- The dangers to the mother and the child
- Effective treatment can be much like the treatment for PMS
- Counseling and further treatment

Postpartum depression is a very complicated illness that is perhaps even more confusing than Premenstrual Syndrome. After all, the arrival of a newborn is generally thought to be one of the happiest events in a woman's life. Why should she be depressed afterwards?

How do you explain someone like Eve P.? At thirty-three, she had a good marriage, had finally gotten pregnant, was overjoyed throughout the pregnancy and ecstatic at the birth of her daughter. Then, two weeks after giving birth, she was tearful, depressed, restless, and unable to sleep. She was afraid to hold or care for her child.

Eve isn't alone. Roughly 10 percent of women experience some depressed feelings, ranging from mild to severe depression.

People frequently do not recognize postpartum depression for what it is, because it does not always occur immediately after childbirth. It can occur weeks, or even months, after delivery.

It is a different illness, but like PMS, postpartum depression is hormonally determined. No woman should blame herself because her healthy, stable personality is transformed into one which is despairing and so estranged from her normal state that she may even have thoughts of harming her baby. Very complicated hormonal shifts occur after childbirth. Some can be devastating.

Women with postpartum depression frequently do blame themselves. It's not uncommon to hear them speaking about their failure as mothers.

In the past, the common treatments for postpartum depression fed right into that sense of guilt. Not knowing any better, psychiatrists assumed that some powerful psychological disturbance was behind PPD. The most common psychiatric diagnosis was: "This woman is having trouble accepting her role as a mother."

What Causes Postpartum Depression?

We really don't know what causes postpartum depression. The major cause is probably the drastic changes in hormone levels postpartum. Progesterone levels during pregnancy can be fifteen to thirty times the peak levels experienced by a nonpregnant woman. After delivery, estrogen and progesterone levels in the body are reduced to insignificant levels, and four other hormones unique to pregnancy disappear completely.

More importantly, one particular hormone, prolactin, rises markedly to prepare the breasts for lactation. Estrogen and progesterone remain low, and the woman does not menstruate. As long as a woman breast-feeds, she will continue to have an elevated prolactin level. But, according to Dr. Katharina Dalton, even women who do not breast-feed continue to have raised prolactin for some weeks—sometimes for as long as two months.

Menstruation will begin again once prolactin levels return to normal. Unfortunately, if a woman has suffered postpartum depression, the return of menstruation will probably also signal the return (or the beginning) of PMS. Dalton's research showed that over 90 percent of the women who suffered a postpartum depression went on to develop Premenstrual Syndrome.

What Does That Mean to You?

The first step is to *anticipate*. Be aware that it is perfectly possible to have other than expected feelings after the birth of your child. Understand that those feelings, if they occur, will be due to underlying hormonal changes and not due to anything wrong with you as a person or a mother. If you already have had PMS, the symptoms will probably lessen—and may even disappear—as your body starts to increase its production of progesterone during pregnancy. But be aware that your PMS is likely to return and act *now* to *prepare* yourself.

If you do develop postpartum depression, establish a positive support network quickly. Make your family aware that you aren't feeling quite up to par and that you may need additional professional help during this difficult period. If the feelings become intense, you would certainly be well advised to seek out such help.

Most mild postpartum depression does not last that long. While it lasts, you may experience a wide variety of feelings including elation, mood swings, and momentary paralyzing despondency. You should share these feelings with your supportive family members and friends so they can help you to make sure things aren't getting out of hand.

WHAT YOU SHOULD PARTICULARLY WATCH FOR

Worsening depression. If you are consistently depressed for more than a week and the depression deepens, *consult your doctor immediately!* Usually your gynecologist will be the first line of help.

Extreme thoughts. If you start having extreme thoughts that really seem like they don't belong in your head, thoughts you have never experienced before—like fleeting thoughts of hurting the child— you must *immediately consult with a knowledgeable psychiatrist* so that your condition can be assessed. In the vast majority of cases, these thoughts are fleeting, but it is best to be prepared and to get help early to prevent a real problem from occurring. Tragedies seldom occur, but make no mistake about it, untreated postpartum depression can be a dangerous situation for the lives of both the mother and the child.

The Mother Who Shopped at Bloomingdales

We always begin by learning whatever we can about the menstrual and hormonal condition of a postpartum woman *before* her pregnancy. This establishes a baseline.

Then we place the woman on exactly the same treatment program as our normal PMS patients. However, if it seems that there is any possible risk to the mother or the child, we immediately institute progesterone treatment and provide constant supervision.

Sometimes progesterone does it! Over the years, we have used natural progesterone as our major treatment intervention in postpartum depression with a very high rate of success. In treating PPD, however, we must be more careful to involve the family and we must monitor the treatment with scrupulous concern because of the sudden mood changes characteristic of this disorder. Above all, every situation needs an individual evaluation of the precise risk to the child.

We recommend the immediate use of progesterone as the first but not the only line of treatment. It can be dramatically effective and lifesaving.

Melissa R. was a great example. Her mother called us and said that her daughter had become paralyzingly depressed since the birth of her baby. "Come in and see us, today," we said. We didn't anticipate that this beautiful young model would arrive escorted by an ambulance attendant. She was barely able to stand, barely able to speak. While we made arrangements for her to be hospitalized, we gave her some progesterone. When Dr. Martorano returned to the waiting room, Melissa and her mother were nowhere in sight. Concerned, he questioned a staff member, who said, "Oh, she was feeling so much better that they went to shop at Bloomingdales. They'll be back in an hour." Few treatments that we'd seen resulted in that dramatic a recovery, but this one did.

Postpartum disorders require a great deal of skill and patience. If there is not immediate improvement, it is important to initiate antidepressant treatment as soon as possible, in addition to maintaining the progesterone treatment.

Finally, if there is any evidence of psychotic thoughts, it may be essential to add an anti-psychotic medication like Haldol® to attack these intrusive, unwanted, and potentially dangerous thoughts.

And Sleep, Of Course

Adequate quantities of good quality nightly sleep are essential to complete recovery. Every effort must be made to ensure it.

You may get your family and friends to share the nighttime duties with regard to the newborn child, so that you can get at least four or five nights of uninterrupted sleep.

You can use a short-term tranquilizer like Ativan® or Centrax® to help restore the full night's sleep, or, if necessary, you can resort to the *short-term* use of a sleeping medication. **But remember, you cannot take medications if you breast feed, unless you have specific approval from your doctor.**

It is absolutely necessary to restore sleep so that your body's physiological processes can return to normal. Not infrequently, this seemingly simple therapeutic intervention will reverse all the painful symptoms of mild postpartum depression.

Counseling If You Need It

Of course, any competent therapist can provide some needed counseling for the mother with postpartum depression. The essential aspect of such preliminary counseling is to teach her to accept the fact that this disorder is physiologic, and there is not something inherently wrong with her. Full realization of the fact will serve to keep her self-respect and self-esteem intact, so that she can more fully enjoy the pleasures of her newborn child.

Together with the medical treatments described, counseling will usually bring a fair measure of success to the treatment of PPD. However, each case is unique, There may be psychological problems and dysfunctional family interactions that make further help advisable. Such therapy is often a good and even necessary addition.

There are a growing number of support and professional help organizations for women suffering from postpartum depression and other postpartum symptoms. The best known and our best resource is Depression After Delivery (DAD), which is headed by Nancy Berchtold and headquartered in Pennsylvania and which can be reached at 215 295-3994.

13

Menopause

THIS CHAPTER WILL SHOW YOU:

- The typical experiences of a menopausal woman
- The choices in postmenopausal hormone supplementation
- Why low progesterone also affects menopausal women
- The importance of avoiding synthetic progesterone in treatment

Menopause can be difficult. Irene A. was typical. A fiftyish successful businesswoman with a harried schedule, she was "Too busy to get better," she confided in us. "But I'm also a mess." And she was.

Irene became increasingly depressed as she approached fifty. It wasn't an easy age for her. Her children had left home, her work was sometimes successful, between her husband and herself there was an increasing irritability—the signs of an aging marriage perhaps. Irene was somewhat startled and somewhat chagrined by her diminished sex drive.

But it was the problems of mental functioning that really shook her. She suffered from occasional short-term memory loss. It seemed to her that her brain was no longer the useful and efficient instrument that it had been.

This sense of personal diminishment peaked after she had two minor auto accidents that she felt had been brought on by a lack of alertness on her part. She became terrified of driving and, occasionally, when her husband or a friend couldn't drop her off, she would miss work.

Irene tied all this to the fact that her periods were now irregular or infrequent. Ask anyone on the street, they would make the correct diagnosis: Irene was going through menopause.

Menopause and the Great Hormone Debate

Menopause is the time when a woman's fertility and monthly menstrual period comes to an end. The process can take anywhere from one year to several years, and it's estimated that in the next two decades nearly forty million women will pass through menopause. Most women experience at least some of the well-known change-of-life symptoms such as hot flashes, dry skin, backaches, depression, and mental confusion. And now, women must also decide whether they want to take hormones to control these symptoms.

A great medical debate has arisen over the benefits versus the perils of taking hormones, especially estrogen, to counteract the effects of menopause. We won't be able to solve that debate in this chapter. Quite apart from its alleviation of some menopausal symptoms, estrogen is beneficial in slowing bone loss and in protecting against some heart disease. Unfortunately, there *is* some evidence (albeit controversial) of a grim negative lurking in the wings: that supplemental estrogen, when taken alone, may increase the risk of certain kinds of cancer, especially cancer of the endometrial lining of the uterus.

This fear of cancer has caused more and more physicians to advocate supplemental progesterone be given concurrently with estrogen to counteract the potentially carcinogenic effects of estrogen, and this type of therapy is commonly called *Biphasal Hormone Replacement Therapy* (BHRT).

If done properly, we think this is a very logical and beneficial development in patient care and *not* just because it will help protect you from cancer. You see, another aspect of menopause, in addition to declining estrogen levels, is the decline in progesterone levels. The emphasis on estrogen-related problems tends to shift attention away from a frequent increase in PMS symptoms due to the abrupt decrease of progesterone that occurs at menopause. There is, for instance, a worsening of hypoglycemia that is marked by some of the more compelling menopausal signs like hot flashes.

Let's Look at Irene Again

Irene complained to her gynecologist of hot flashes, irritability, painful vaginal dryness during intercourse, bloating, and some memory loss. Her gynecologist had guided her through two pregnancies and several mammograms for fibrocystic disease, and he certainly wanted to ward off the possible detrimental effects of menopause including osteoporosis. He carefully discusses with Irene the pros and cons of estrogen therapy versus Biphasal Hormone Replacement Therapy. She opted for BHRT. Her doctor then prescribed Premarin® (the form of estrogen that is most commonly used) and *medroxy progesterone*, the synthetic progesterone that is generally used in BHRT.

Irene began the treatment, and, as the estrogen kicked in, enjoyed marked improvement. Her hot flashes stopped almost completely. She enjoyed renewed sexual interest coupled with increased lubrication. Things were looking up!

Unfortunately, not for long. Irene became yet another victim of the American pharmaceutical industry's $5 billion-a-year advertising budget directed toward convincing doctors to use drugs like synthetic progesterone.

The synthetic progesterone has been added to oppose estrogen's carcinogenic effects, and it did, but it also did much else besides. Synthetic progesterone competes for the same receptor sites as natural progesterone. Thus it deprived Irene of the beneficial effects of natural progesterone. She gained ten pounds and suffered painfully tender breasts and abdominal bloating.

The discomfort went on until she wondered if she should stop her BHRT. And her occasional mental confusion and memory loss had now grown more than occasional and gave her trouble at work.

"I can't remember a thing," says Irene, "maybe I have Alzheimer's."

Do You Know the Answer?

We suspect that by this point in the book you probably know the answer to Irene's problems. Right! It's blood glucose—the only nutrient that the brain uses as fuel—that Irene was short on. Her underlying PMS, which, prior to menopause, had never been serious enough to cause her real problems or make her seek medical care, started to get worse as her progesterone levels declined during the onset of menopause.

These lower progesterone levels aggravated a previously rather mild tendency toward low blood sugar. Consequently, Irene experienced the signs of mental confusion that we first described.

The reason those problems got worse is that the Biphasal Hormone Replacement Therapy, which correctly used estrogen to treat Irene's hot flashes and vaginal dryness, *incorrectly* used *synthetic progesterone* to offset the estrogen. Irene's natural supply of progesterone was being driven down even further by this synthetic competitor and consequently her brain problems were getting worse daily.

When Irene came to PMS Medical, we kept her on estrogen but replaced the synthetic with natural progesterone in its oral micronized form. As her blood sugar levels came back to normal, she noticed an immediate improvement in her thinking, and her short-term memory loss disappeared completely.

Interestingly, Irene was so startled by this immediate clinical improvement that she questioned it. So we sent her over to our collaborative laboratories at the New York Center for Brain Study and there they did brain mapping (computerized electroencephalography) while giving Irene a dose of oral progesterone. Immediate improvements in her vigilance and in the cognitive aspects of her brain function were demonstrated on the brain maps by clear changes in electrical functioning. The change was shown to be statistically significant when checked out against the exhaustive data base which we have collected from CEEG centers around the world. It's possible to demonstrate directly, through brain mapped improvements in cerebral function, that progesterone is working.

A Final Word on Menopause

The final word on menopause—for now—is that for women with serious menopausal symptoms or serious fears of heart disease and osteoporosis, Biphasal Hormone Replacement Therapy is well worth considering. But if you use BHRT work to convince your physician that a synthetic form of progesterone is not "just the same" as natural progesterone. Believe us, it isn't.

If you are already on synthetic progesterone and aren't experiencing any side effects, you should probably continue just as you are. But continue to watch for the appearance of side effects.

If you *are* experiencing side effects, then consider changing to natural progesterone. Approach your doctor about making the change. With any luck, he will have an open mind. But, if he doesn't and the problems continue, then consider consulting with someone more experienced with the natural form of progesterone.

Interlude

Fluid Retention

Another problem that's as familiar to premenstrual women as breathing is fluid retention. It can certainly be one of the most painful and burdensome aspects of Premenstrual Syndrome and there's a lot you can do to control it. In the last chapter we looked at the relationship between fluid retention and dysmennorrhea. Now let's look at it in relation to PMS.

When we speak of breast tenderness, abdominal bloating, weight gain, most women can think back to at least some personal experiences in these areas. Certainly sodium and fluid retention can be a weighty problem. We have seen a famous actress who had to change her costume size not once but *twice* during one night's performance of a play on account of bloating. Some women gain incredible amounts of weight premenstrually—as much as ten or even fifteen pounds monthly. That's much the same as tying three five pound bags of sugar around your waist for two weeks a month.

The female hormone estrogen causes the body to store salt and often causes women to crave salt. This is a double jeopardy since salt retains body fluids and, therefore, to a woman predisposed by her menstrual cycle to fluid retention, excess salt is the short road to bloatedness. Yet, when women's estrogen levels are high, they often find themselves eating salty foods and salting everything else that they eat. It's a very bad move. This is one craving that must be resisted. It's also worth remembering that in some people high salt consumption can lead to high blood pressure.

The Diuretic Nonsolution—And One Exception

Most women, desperate to reduce swelling and not wanting to suffer such distress, turn to diuretics for help. Unfortunately, diuretics are not the best solution and shouldn't be used at first because they invariably produce side effects. Their prolonged use can cause fatigue due to the loss of potassium from the body. And though they do remove fluid, they do nothing at all to help with the other symptoms of PMS. Sadder still, if you take them long enough, your body restabilizes itself and learns to resist the diuretics.

The major exception to our disapproval of diuretics is a drug called *spironolactone*. A different type of diuretic, it exerts its special effects on renin, aldosterone, and angiostensin—adrenal hormones that are collectively called the aldosterone system—which appear to increase premenstrually. These adrenal hormones are believed to cause fluid retention, and spironolactone seems able to counterbalance their undesirable effects.

Therefore, we sometimes recommend spironolactone when we see a severe symptom, such as excruciating breast tenderness, that is not relieved by our usual program. When used properly, this diuretic causes little of the potassium loss associated with other diuretics. However, spironolactone has to be prescribed and monitored by your physician.

A Simpler, More Effective Solution

The first and easiest way of treating fluid retention is to eliminate salt from your diet. (Say goodbye to pickles!) Examine your entire diet for substances that contain salt. Use the list on pages 165–167. Remember that most canned and frozen foods are salted to enhance flavor. Look for sodium (the chemical name for salt) on the labels of the food you buy.

Remember—plan to prevent fluid retention, which is much easier to accomplish than it is to relieve it.

Here are five other steps that can help:

1. Try to incorporate foods into your diet that have natural diuretic properties such as strawberries and parsley.
2. Use 500 mg. capsules of Evening Primrose Oil (up to six a day); this substance is rich in linoleic acid, one of the body's essential fatty acids, and promising research both in this country and in England suggests it can help limit fluid retention.
3. Don't restrict your consumption of fluids. The idea that this will work to prevent fluid retention is a common myth. Restricting fluids causes dehydration and other problems.
4. Exercise regularly and aerobically. Your fatty tissues are your fluid-retaining tissues, and the more you replace fat with muscle, the less likely you are to be bothered by fluid retention.
5. When indicated, ask your doctor to use natural progesterone to assist your body in naturally eliminating excess fluid.

Most women who take these steps find that fluid retention becomes a relatively minor part of their menstrual cycle. You're gaining more of a handle on your PMS. Now keep up the good work!

Note: If you have swelling/bloating which persists throughout the month, this could indicate a serious medical problem. Let your menstrual calendar be your guide. Consult a doctor if it's not relieved by our five-step plan.

THE PMS
NUTRITIONAL
TREATMENT PLAN

14

Changing Your Life

THIS CHAPTER WILL SHOW YOU:

- The life-style changes that will help you to treat your PMS symptoms
- Specific tips for making these changes
- The importance of keeping records
- How to find out when you ovulate

Almost every aspect of your treatment for PMS will require that you make changes in your present life-style. We know that it can be difficult to make these changes, so this chapter is designed to assist you in making the process of change easier.

The changes we'll be asking you to make involve many of the following areas:

1. *Observing and charting*: daily temperature, daily symptoms, occurrence and menstruation, food and beverages consumed—both amount and time of consumption.
2. *Making nutritional changes*: reducing carbohydrates and refined sugar, reducing sodium, increasing protein and fat intake, eating at least six small meals a day, taking recommended vitamin and mineral supplements.
3. *Rescheduling your activities* to create less stress at times when you have symptoms. This includes: moving appointments (when possible) to a symptom-free period; planning and making low-sodium and low-sugar meals ahead of time, so that you won't have to bother when you have the symptoms; and taking brief rests during the days you feel poorly.

4. *Implementing an exercise regimen* to help fine tune your metabolism, increase your physical stamina, reduce stress, aid in deterring fluid retention, and facilitate weight maintenance or weight loss.
5. *Using relaxation exercises* at appropriate times.
6. *Using cognitive restructuring* to change negative thoughts.

At first, you may find this list of changes a bit overwhelming. You will need to set priorities. Read over the breakdown of symptoms in chapter 2. When you have determined what seems to be contributing to your symptoms, you'll have a good idea of where to begin making changes. For example, if fatigue is the symptom that troubles you most, you'll want to begin eating six small meals, taking brief rests, and beginning some type of aerobic exercise. You might also want to prepare meals in advance to lighten your work load on the days when you feel fatigue.

It's a good idea to keep track of each change you make. This way you'll be able to evaluate the effectiveness of the change, and you'll also be able to see your progress.

How To Make Changes

Like anything else, making life-style changes is easier if you plan ahead.

- Make a list of the changes you need to make.
- Arrange the items on the list in order of their importance to you.
- Set a time frame for making each change.
- Discuss your plans with a family member or close friend who can encourage you.
- Check yourself at the end of each week to evaluate how well you're sticking to your plan.
- Give yourself a reward for completing your weekly plan properly—a movie, bath oil, something small, but a tangible gift from you to you.

Don't become discouraged if you run into difficulty reaching your goal. Make your goal realistic; plan only a few changes each week so as not to make it too difficult to reach your goals. The treatment plan works only when you work with it.

Specific Suggestions for Change

OBSERVING AND CHARTING

Keep your menstrual calendar and your thermometer on your nightstand so that they will be handy for recording in the morning and at the end of the day.

Tape a sheet of paper and a pencil to the wall in the bathroom so that you can record your weight after urinating in the morning.

Fill out your menstrual calendar each day. If you try to rely on memory, you may forget an important item of information. Chart your symptoms.

It is essential that you keep complete records; this way you will have compelling evidence and specific data if you should need professional assistance.

It's important to remember that you must keep daily records for at least two consecutive months. The records also help you stay on track and monitor your successes.

NUTRITIONAL CHANGES

Read the labels on the foods you buy.

Have appropriate foods and snacks readily available.

Put the salt away.

Keep alternatives to salt at hand.

Carry a small bag of dried fruit and nuts in your purse.

Prepare ahead and freeze a few low-salt meals for days when you'll expect to have symptoms.

When you feel a craving for a specific kind of food, make certain that it is sugar- and salt-free.

Plan on having acceptable substitute foods on hand for when you get a craving. (You might decide to eat a banana or peanut butter and rice crackers when you feel a chocolate craving.)

If you need to take vitamins and/or minerals during the day, be sure to carry them with you. Have a plan in mind for eating less at meal times so that you'll be able to eat six small meals without gaining weight.

Don't skip any meals!

RESCHEDULING

Learn to identify the activities and events that regularly cause you the most stress. Plan to do as few of these stressful things as possible on the days when you'll have symptoms.

Plan to do your more difficult or demanding work when you expect to be symptom-free.

If you find that you're having a difficult day unexpectedly, try to reschedule some of your activities for a better time. It's wiser to reschedule than to have troubling symptoms return.

See if you can enlist the help of a family member, coworker, or friend to give a little help on your difficult days.

If you have small children, see if you can find a friend who is willing to babysit for you on your worst days, in return for caring for her children at a time when you are not premenstrual.

If you are a working person, try to keep your work schedule more flexible on the days when you are premenstrual.

Plan to shop and do other heavy chores on those days when you are symptom-free.

EXERCISE

Find an *aerobic exercise* you enjoy, such as walking, jogging, biking. (Remember "aerobic" refers to measurable effect on heart rate and respiration.)

Look into exercise tapes, which may make it easier for you to get started.

Bear in mind the importance of warming up and cooling down in any good exercise program; these help prevent injury.

Begin your exercise on the day that your menstruation subsides. This way you'll follow your program for at least a week before you experience any symptoms that might make it difficult for you to stick with it.

Try to get your exercise time in before the very end of the day when you might be too tired to exercise.

Using Basal Body Temperature to Determine Ovulation

It is very important to determine the exact day in your cycle when you ovulate (when your ovary releases the egg for its journey down the fallopian tube towards the uterus). The symptoms of PMS generally occur between ovulation and menstruation. Charting the relationship between the day you ovulate and the onset of the various symptoms you experience can assist you in preparing for an eventually evaluating the effects of the treatment plan.

Ovulation coincides with the production by the ovary of progesterone. Among its other effects, progesterone makes its presence known by its significant upward effect on the Basal Body Temperature (BTT), the normal body temperature of a healthy person immediately upon awakening after a restful night's sleep.

The elevation in temperature, which will be sustained until ovarian progesterone secretion stops and menstruation follows, may range from a half to a full degree farenheit. Provided no other illness is present, the charting of several monthly cycles of your daily BBT should plainly identify your day of ovulation and its relationship to your symptoms.

HOW TO TAKE YOUR BBT

Buy a thermometer (available at any pharmacy). We recommend you use a rectal thermometer because rectal temperature is the most accurate. Coating the thermometer with a lubricant (such as

K-Y Jelly) will make it easier to insert. However, if you start your observations with an oral thermometer, don't switch.

Take your temperature immediately upon awakening, every day. Postpone any activity, including smoking, eating, drinking, or urinating, until you have taken your temperature, as it may tend to raise your temperature. Relax in the knowledge that you are doing something good for yourself.

After a full five minutes by the clock, read the thermometer.

Other Signs of Ovulation

A milky (clear to white), gel-like discharge will be seen for two to three days at ovulation. You may also experience a small sharp pain in your lower abdomen (at the ovaries). This pain, however, alternates sides from month to month as ovulation does, and is sometimes less severe on one side than the other, making it less reliable for charting.

15

Nutritional Therapy for PMS

THIS CHAPTER WILL SHOW YOU:

- How to keep your blood sugar level from dropping to the critical symptom level
- How to reduce sodium in your diet
- The use of vitamins and minerals in treating PMS
- The importance of Evening Primrose Oil

The key to controlling your PMS is in *scheduling* the proper diet. It is absolutely essential that you keep an eating schedule in your premenstrual time and never go more than two to three hours without eating some small amount of recommended foods.

The way to start is by writing down an accurate daily record of exactly what you eat and the exact times you eat it. A recurrence of symptoms can frequently be accounted for only by going over the diet record and finding a hidden breakdown in the recommended procedures.

Keeping an accurate daily record of exactly what you eat and drink is absolutely crucial in controlling PMS.

Our experience indicates the best way to keep an accurate record is to carry a small pocket-sized notebook with you at all times. Be careful to note anything you eat and drink and with special attention to snacks, which are often the most neglected entries in the record. Be sure to record the *exact time* you eat.

There are several major psychological abnormalities associated with PMS that frequently can be *completely* corrected simply

Sample Food Journal, Pretreatment			
Time	Food	Drink	Symptoms
Morning 8:30 A.M.	muffin	coffee, o.j.	
10:30 A.M.		coffee	
Afternoon 1:30 P.M.	salad with Russian dressing	coke	weakness
4:30 P.M.	no meal		headache
Evening 7:30 P.M.	hamburger, f.f.	water	dizziness & fatigue
10:30 P.M.	no meal (asleep)		

by nutritional treatment. It is important for you to understand the background of these changes in order to maintain the proper diet.

The two most important abnormalities associated with PMS are: relative hypoglycemia, which may appear only premenstrually and is related to a relative lack of progesterone; and increased salt retention causing water retention throughout the body.

A Review of Hypoglycemia

As you know, glucose is the only nutrient utilized by the brain. Therefore, relatively minor changes in it will cause distressing symptoms.

All sugars fall into one of three categories. *Monosaccharides* are single sugars such as glucose (blood sugar; fructose or fruit sugar; and galactose or milk sugar). Glucose is either oxidized (burned) by the cells in our bodies to provide them with energy, or converted into glycogen and stored in the liver for use later on.

Disaccharides are two sugar molecules attached to one another. Sucrose, the sugar found in table sugar or sugar cane, and maltose, which is present in barley and honey, are both disaccharides. These and all other dissacharides are not directly absorbed by the blood stream, but must be acted upon by digestive enzymes. The enzymes break them down into simple sugars, glucose and fructose, which are in turn absorbed into the blood stream or converted into glycogen and stored in the liver.

Polysaccharides are many sugars linked together. This category includes starch, dextrose, cellulose, and glycogen.

Decreased blood sugar first affects the circulatory system. The heart automatically reacts as the body attempts to restore balance to the system. This reaction may result in an immediately rapid and irregular pulse with palpitations and breathing difficulties.

How to Keep Your Blood Sugar Level from Dropping to the Symptom Level

To keep your blood sugar level from dropping to a level where it will cause problems, we recommend the following:

1. *Eat three daily meals with three mini meals (snacks) in between.* **Do not fast or skip meals.** You want to feed your body a constant supply of food that it can convert to glucose. Don't go longer than three hours without eating, and stick to the recommended foods.
2. *Eat complex carbohydrate and high protein foods (see list below).* These are easily converted to glucose over a long time period, providing the body with a constant supply of glucose for the bloodstream. These complex carbohydrates also contain vitamins, minerals, and fiber that have been processed out of refined foods. The quality of foods is an important factor to be taken into account as you plan your diet.

3. *Avoid simple carbohydrates.* Simple carbohydrates, such as refined sugars and flours, are unhealthy because these foods require little or no digestion to enter the bloodstream. The levels of glucose in the bloodstream, which these foods have so swiftly supplied, is lowered just as swiftly by insulin. The reduction is so severe, your body soon finds itself reacting to the starvation level of blood sugar.

4. *Avoid caffeine and alcohol.* These foods adversely affect the free sugars in the blood, causing abnormal rises and falls in blood sugar.

Plan your diet to include these foods instead:

COMPLEX CARBOHYDRATES AND HIGH-PROTEIN, LOW-FAT FOODS

- *Grains.* Whole wheat breads and rolls, whole grain breads (rye and pumpernickel), pita bread, corn tortillas, sugar-free cereals, sprouted wheat berries, brown rice, and other grain foods.
- *Vegetables.* Preferably steamed, grilled, or raw; avoid overcooking.
- *Fruits and fruit juices.* Preferably fresh, if canned or frozen, eat only those without added sweeteners. Drink only very diluted cranberry or apple juice. Avoid citrus fruit juices.
- *Dairy products.* Drink only skim milk, and stick to low-sodium, low-fat cheese; low-sodium, low-fat cottage cheese; and unsalted butter or margarine in small amounts.
- *Meat, fish, and poultry.* Eat only lean meats, chicken, tuna, and other fish.

Avoid: Sugar, citrus juices, alcohol, fructose, white flour, white rice, cake, carob, candy, cookies, soft drinks, ice cream, sherbet, pastries, pies, puddings, Jello®, jelly or marmalade, honey, artificial sweeteners, white bread, and other highly refined foods.

USE HIGH-PROTEIN, COMPLEX-CARBOHYDRATE SNACKS FOR "MINI MEALS"

- Peanut butter sandwich, preferably made with natural, un-sweetened peanut butter and *no jelly*
- Assorted raw, salt-free nuts mixed with a small amount of raisins
- Plain low-calorie yogurt with fresh fruit, such as banana
- Cold cereal with low-calorie milk
- Rice crackers with low-sodium cheese
- Low-sodium cheese and fresh fruit, such as apple
- Peanut butter on brown rice crackers
- Low-fat or skim milk and sugar-free graham crackers
- Low-sodium cottage cheese and fruit

Sodium and PMS

Sodium is needed in the blood at the proper concentration to provide our tissues with adequate levels of water. Excess sodium retention and secondary water retention can produce many PMS symptoms including abdominal bloating, breast tenderness and swelling, dizziness, and backache.

Sodium and water are handled similarly by the major chemical regulators of our bodies, the kidneys. If sodium is excreted, water is also lost in the urine. If sodium is retained—or more correctly, reabsorbed from the outgoing urine—water is also retained.

Several physiological events that occur between ovulation and menses can create abnormal sodium and water retention. Just after ovulation, progesterone secretion begins and increases dramatically until one week before menses, when—just as dramatically—it drops off to zero. The progesterone is then broken down into two byproducts that exert strong sodium- and water-retaining effects on the kidneys. The stress experienced during this phase by women with PMS triggers the release of more aldosterone and of a more powerful water-retaining hormone called antidiuretic hormone, which also causes fluid retention.

Water retention results in swollen and tender breasts, swelling of the abdomen, weight gain, less frequent urination, swollen ankles, feet, and hands. Fluids also collect in areas where the tissues are incapable of stretching to accommodate the excess body fluids. Such areas are the skull, behind the eye, the labyrinth of the inner ear, the discs between the vertebrae and the spine, and the carpal nerve tunnel of the wrists. Stretching of these areas frequently causes migraines, dizziness, backache, and numbness in the extremities.

If you conscientiously limit your salt intake, you will soon experience a welcome relief in premenstrual bloating and painful tissue swelling.

How to Reduce Sodium in Your Diet

Here are some helpful hints:

- Remove salt shakers from table and stove.
- Never add salt before tasting food you eat.
- Don't buy salted snacks.
- Stock up on salt-free snacks.
- Don't use salt in cooking.
- Keep sliced, ready-to eat vegetables in refrigerator.
- Have fresh fruit available.
- Learn to read labels on food before you buy it.
- Experiment with spices to add flavor to foods.
- Try using herbs as seasoning.
- Learn to make your own salt-free mayonnaise and catsup.
- Keep lemon juice or vinegar handy to use in flavoring foods.
- Steaming vegetables instead of boiling will retain their natural flavor.
- Avoid processed foods, particularly canned and frozen foods. Salted dips are often used to prepare vegetables for freezing.

Salt is also added in alarming quantities to canned foods in order to enhance the flavor lost in over-processing.

Don't feel guilty for depriving your family members of salt. The amount of sodium consumed by the average person in the United States is ten to twenty times higher than is required for health. Since high blood pressure can be a side effect of a high-salt diet, you are helping to prevent illness by placing the entire family on a restricted sodium diet. Eventually your taste accommodates and you simply won't want or miss it.

WHAT ABOUT THE NEED TO REPLACE SALT AFTER STRENUOUS WORK OR EXERCISE?

Current research seems to indicate that after strenuous exercise it is more important to replace lost fluid and lost potassium than lost salt. The body is unable to store potassium but it does have reserves of sodium. If you need to replace sodium, try a 4 oz. serving of salted tomato juice (all regular tomato juice is salted) and note any bloating for 24 hours. In future, increase or decrease the serving size by 1 to 2 oz. depending on your observations.

Adjust Your Diet to Include These Low-Sodium Foods

Cereals

Cream of Wheat® (regular)
Ralston® (instant and regular)
Puffed rice
Rolled oats
Wheatena®
Puffed wheat
Shredded wheat

Crackers

Matzoh, unsalted plain
Whole rice wafers

Other Cereal Products

Pasta (fresh or enriched are the best)
Egg noodles
Rice (brown or wild)

Fruits (Fresh)

Apples
Apricots, fresh or dried
Bananas
Blackberries
Blueberries
Cherries
Dates
Figs, fresh or dried
Grapefruits
Lemons
Oranges
Peaches
Pears
Pineapples
Plums
Prunes
Raspberries
Tangerines
Watermelon

Vegetables (Fresh)

Asparagus
Beans
Broccoli
Brussel sprouts
Cabbage
Cauliflower
Corn

Lettuce
Mushrooms
Okra
Onions
Peas
Peppers, green
Potatoes
Radishes
Squash
Sweet potatoes
Tomatoes
Turnips, yellow
Turnip greens

Meats, Fish, Poultry[2]

Beef, lean
Chicken (average, light, and dark)
Codfish
Halibut
Lamb
Liver
Salmon, canned in water, unsalted
Tuna, canned in water, unsalted

Avoid the Following High-Sodium Foods

Vegetables

Frozen peas
Frozen lima beans
Artichokes
Beet greens
Beets
Celery

---

[2]Contains less than 100 mgs. of sodium per 3 ½ serving.

Kale
Mustard greens
Sauerkraut
Spinach
Chard
White turnips

Fish

Anchovies
Canned fish
Caviar
Clams
Crabs
Herring
Lobster
Salted fish
Sardines
Shellfish
Shrimp
Scallops

Baked Goods

Processed breads (examine the label carefully)
Cakes
Most cereals
Crackers
Potato chips
Pretzels
Salted popcorn

Vitamins and PMS

Vitamins are organic compounds that are required in minute quantities to serve as catalysts in the processes that turn food into energy and living tissue.

We cannot replace the loss of vitamins by synthesizing them in our bodies. We must obtain them from the environment. A vitamin deficiency causes a reduction in the rate of the metabolic process in which it is involved. There are two main groups of vitamins:

The fat-soluble vitamins (A, D, E, and K)

The water-soluble vitamins (B Complex, C)

Vitamin B_6 (*pyridoxine*) has been intimately linked to brain functions. It is an essential brain cell nutrient. B_6 also plays an important role in the metabolism of amino acids in our bodies and is required in sufficient quantities before our bodies can properly produce estrogen and progesterone.

In some women, the lack of vitamin B_6 has a harmful effect on the chemical pathways in the hypothalamus and the pituitary. A B_6 deficiency causes a decrease in the production of dopamine; dopamine inhibits the production of prolactin. If dopamine is not present in proper amounts, the uninhibited prolactin is, therefore, present in higher than normal amounts, this results in adverse affects on the ovaries, on the breasts, and possibly on the fluid balance. A deficiency in B_6 can also result in lowered serotonin levels which have been found to induce depression.

The use of B_6 is one of the mildest and simplest treatments for PMS. Because it is a water-soluble vitamin, excess is not stored in your body but is freely excreted in the urine.

We recommend you start with a 50 mg. dose a day and increase it to a maximum of 150 mgs. per day until you notice results. Reports indicate that the therapeutic effect of B_6 is noticed only if you have reached the correct level. So don't be discouraged if you don't see results immediately. The only common side effect is that high doses may cause a mild gastric acidity. It is commonly recommended that B_6 therapy be continued for a minimum of nine months.

When B_6 is taken in high doses, it should always be taken in conjunction with other B vitamins because it tends to deplete the other B vitamins. We recommend that you take B_6 in the form of a B-complex vitamin in order to assure you are getting the proper amounts of all the B vitamins. If B_6 helps you may continue taking it throughout the month. **Caffeine, mineral oil, and alcohol are**

Foods That Are Rich in Vitamin B_6

Fresh meats, especially liver, kidney, and beef
Wheat, bran, and wholemeal bread
Fresh vegetables, especially cabbage
Brown rice
Brewer's yeast
Milk and eggs

Processes and Substances That Decrease Levels of B_6 in the Body

Canning
Roasting or stewing meat
Food-processing techniques
Sleeping pills
Caffeine
Water
Sulfa drugs
Alcohol
Estrogen
Excessively stored food

---

known antagonists to the B vitamins and should be minimized or totally avoided in the PMS diet.

Vitamin A has also been reported to relieve some PMS symptoms. Believed to have a diuretic effect, it is said to alleviate abdominal bloating, swollen breasts, and other tissues. It has also been known to combat stress and fatigue.

Consult with your doctor, before going on any fat-soluble vitamin therapy (Vitamins A, D, E, and K). Taken in high doses, such vitamins can be toxic.

Foods That Are Rich in Vitamin A

Green and yellow vegetables
Fruit, especially yellow fruits
Dairy products
Egg yolk
Carrots
Liver

Minerals and PMS

It has been established that calcium, magnesium, and potassium play a vital role in the normal biochemistry of the neuromuscular system. Their presence in sufficient quantities in and around the brain, nerve, and muscle cells are required if these organs are to function properly.

In a study reported in the November 1981 issue of *The American Journal of Clinical Nutrition*, women with PMS symptoms were shown to have an intracellular magnesium level significantly lower than women without these symptoms.

CLINICAL CLUE

Chocolate Cravings

We have found that chocolate cravings are often related to *magnesium deficiency*. These cravings often disappear with the regular use of mineral supplements that include replacement levels of magnesium.

Calcium-rich Foods

Dairy products: skim milk, low-sodium, cheeses, yogurt
Dark green and yellow vegetables: zucchini, squash, broccoli, asparagus—preferably cooked until tender in as little water as possible, steamed or eaten raw. (Unsweetened vegetable juices may be used to replace a cooked vegetable or as a between-meal snack.)

Magnesium-rich Foods

Whole grain breads and cereals
Fresh green vegetables
Peanut butter

Potassium-rich Foods

All fresh fruits (but not juices) especially oranges, bananas, tomatoes, and apricots.

Potassium levels drop during the premenstrual period when sodium and water are being retained. It is excreted in larger than usual amounts in the urine.

What all this means is that you should be sure to include adequate intake of these minerals in your diet.

Your Vitamin Lineup

It will be helpful to know what a useful PMS vitamin and mineral supplement should contain. Many of the following requirements will be met if you eat a healthy diet, but it will not hurt to also take them in supplement form to be sure you obtain what's needed. We recommend that you get the following daily amounts:

Vitamin A—10,000 to 15,000 mgs.
B complex (riboflavin, niacin, thiamine)—25 to 50 mgs.

B_6—50 to 150 mgs.
Vitamin E—100 to 600 I.U.
Calcium—100 to 150 mgs.
Magnesium—200 to 300 mgs.
Zinc—25 mgs.
Chromium—100 mgs.
Vitamin C—250 to 1500 mgs.
Vitamin D—100 mgs. (should not be taken in larger doses)

To make life simpler for our patients, we generally recommend that they take a vitamin specifically formulated for PMS. The one that we usually recommend is called Procycle®. It contains all the vitamins and minerals needed for PMS therapy. We recommend 3 to 6 tablets a day, depending on your needs. It can be ordered directly from Madison Pharmacy (1-800-558-7046) in Wisconsin.

A Miracle Molecule: Evening Primrose Oil

Over the past decade, a family of hormone-like substances known as *prostaglandins* have been shown to have great potential in the relief of such diverse ailments as high blood pressure, arthritis, menstrual cramps, and other medical disorders.

The most potent and intensely studied prostaglandins are made from vitamin-like substances called *essential fatty acids*. These fatty acids are like the essential amino acids in that they cannot be manufactured by the body and need to be provided in the diet.

One of the most important and essential fatty acids is *cis-linoleic acid* which is converted to *gamma-lineolic acid* (GLA). GLA is required by the body for the production of the prostaglandin PGE I. PGE I, called by researchers a *miracle molecule*, is one of the most critical prostaglandins.

If not enough GLA is available, then PGE I can't be produced in adequate amounts. Since you can't ingest PGE I because it is destroyed in the digestive process, it is necessary to increase the dietary supply of GLA. **Evening Primrose Oil is the only substantial source of PGE I that can be ingested.**

The use of Evening Primrose Oil to increase the PGE I has been very effective in treating women with severe Premenstrual Syndrome. While it is increasingly difficult to obtain because of possible restrictions, we have found it to be of great value. It has been especially helpful to those patients with severe breast tenderness and swelling.

One theory for the effectiveness of Evening Primrose Oil in some women is that a shortage of essential fatty acids leads to an excess of prolactin, the hormone that produces breast milk and can also cause changes in mood and fluid metabolism. We usually recommend taking 3 to 6 capsules of Evening Primrose Oil every day.

Sample Diet

Our patients frequently request meal plans. The best meal plan is the one you work out yourself, based on the principles outlined in this book, the foods you like, and your budget.

Here is a sample working model:

BREAKFAST	1	slice whole wheat toast (or sugar-free, low-fat muffin)
	2	teaspoons margarine
	1	cup coffee (preferably decaffeinated)
MID-MORNING	4	oz. plain yogurt with or without banana
LUNCH	3	oz. turkey (low-salt)
	2	slices whole wheat bread
	1	medium-size raw carrot
	1	medium-size apple
	1	cup skim milk
MID-AFTERNOON	1	oz. peanut butter
	2	rice crackers

DINNER	5 oz. baked chicken
	½ cup rice pilaf
	½ cup green beans with one teaspoon margarine
	1 cup shredded lettuce, dressed with 2 teaspoons olive oil and vinegar or lemon juice to taste
	½ cantaloupe
EVENING	3 oz. low-fat cottage cheese
	1 piece toast or rye cracker

Don't forget your vitamins, minerals, and Evening Primrose Oil. These should be taken throughout the month.

Remember to record the times and amounts of your meals and snacks; never go more than three hours without eating (to prevent your blood sugar from dropping too low). While this is absolutely necessary premenstrually, most women report feeling even better if they follow this regime *all month long.*

Remember to check the labels on all canned, bottled, and boxed foods. Many of these products contain *hidden sugars.* You may be surprised to discover that the following have sugar: ketchup, tomato sauce, relish, canned corn, frozen pizza, and most cold cereals. This is only a partial list of such foods.

Remember to:

- Eat three daily meals with three mini-meals in-between (eat six times a day premenstrually).
- Eat complex carbohydrates and high protein meals.
- Avoid fasting or skipping meals.
- Avoid simple carbohydrates and refined foods.
- Avoid caffeine.
- Avoid alcohol and citrus juice entirely.
- Stay on this diet to take the vitamins even if you are on natural progesterone.
- Always take your vitamin supplements and Evening Primrose Oil *with meals.*

Will I Gain Weight?

You needn't fear weight gain on this program. You shouldn't be taking in more calories—rather you'll be fueling your body more regularly and efficiently. Here's how to do this:

Take the number of calories needed to maintain your weight. Let's say that number is 1,500. Divide by 6. That gives you 250 calories per meal. You have some flexibility, but no snack should be less than 100 calories and no meal should exceed 500 calories.

A good breakdown of this would be:

30 % protein
20 % fat
50 % carbohydrate

At the 1,500 level, that would translate into 450 calories of protein, 300 calories of fat, and 750 calories of carbohydrate. Women with PMS should not take in fewer than 1200 calories a day. With recommended aerobic exercise and the right foods, women do not experience weight gain on this diet.

You'll certainly have noticed how often we stress the importance of eating frequent small meals during the premenstrual period of the month. Your increased sensitivity to any drop in low blood sugar during that time makes it imperative that you stick to this rule. Allowing your blood sugar level to start falling because of a short period of relative fasting is simply a very risky thing to do.

16

Exercise Therapy for PMS

THIS CHAPTER WILL SHOW YOU:

- How regular aerobic exercise brings about changes to your body
- How much exercise is the right amount
- The importance of warming up and cooling down
- How many calories you burn doing your favorite exercise

Regular aerobic exercise is a vital and effective component of our treatment plan. We'll tell you why and how in just a moment. But first, consider the physiological effects of exercise.

All mammals (except those in captivity), including human beings, exercise regularly as an integral part of staying alive. Over the past two decades, even most zoos have come to realize that their animals need room to exercise to stay healthy and happy. Unfortunately, this realization has not come to many humans. You're probably all too familiar with the term "couch potato". But it's not only TV-watching that keeps us immobile. Many of us in the high-tech era have work that confines us to a sitting position most of the day.

The physiological evolution of the human is far, far behind the intellectual and social evolution. Remember the fight-or-flight response and how often it is inappropriately fired in women with PMS? You know that frequent tension, irritability, and anxiety are a part of the picture. Most of you have experienced the pain of stiff muscles, aching joints, headaches, low back pain and uncomfortable bloating, particularly in the lower parts of your bodies. These are some of the discomforts that routine aerobic exercise can help to alleviate for you.

Here are seven compelling reasons to put exercise into your program. Regular aerobic exercise:

1. boosts your metabolism and helps your body to burn fuel (food) more effectively;
2. produces real biochemical changes that relax muscles and elevate mood;
3. increases muscle density—the ratio of muscle to fatty tissue—that leads to increased energy, stamina, and an increase feeling of physical competence and physical attractiveness;
4. decreases psychological tension and relieves some anxiety;
5. improves functioning of your gastrointestinal tract;
6. improves sleep; and
7. helps to prevent the bodily signs of aging.

Regular Aerobic Exercise Brings About Changes in Your Body

Regular aerobic exercise (twenty-five minutes a day, five days a week) helps the body to become a more efficient fuel-burning engine. This is very important in PMS because optimizing your metabolism will help you to convert glucose to glycogen and vice versa. This will help you to control episodes of low blood sugar.

It's well known now that those who exercise aerobically and regularly report feeling an exercise "high." This is not a psychological effect alone. During and after this kind of exercise the body releases endorphins, chemicals that decrease pain and enhance mood.

Many of the physical complaints of PMS can be relieved or diminished by exercise. These include painful muscles and joints, tension headaches, low back pain, lower body bloating, and the tiredness and irritability that are due to an uncomfortable body.

In addition, any of you who have successfully put a regular exercise program into place in the past will recall that you eventually feel stronger and more physically competent. You begin to look forward to seeing how you can increase your skills.

And let's face it, it's a real boost to our self-esteem to look into the mirror and see the positive physical effects of regular exercise. We look more attractive to ourselves and we feel encouraged when others compliment us on our new figure.

Much of what people mean when they complain of "tension" has to do with body sensations caused by muscles that are not worked properly. The muscles that move and support our bones are called skeletal muscles. They are designed to be used regularly. When you exercise, you alternately stretch and contract groups of muscles. This helps to prevent or relieve the painful sensations that result from unconsciously tensing muscles as a result of anxiety, pain, or holding one position for too long.

If you are anxious, aerobic exercise helps to alter your physiology so as to relieve the by-products and symptoms of anxiety. When you are anxious you usually impose controlled "fleeing" and turn off the fight-or-flight response by using up adrenalin and other chemicals. Also when you exercise in your target aerobic range, you prevent the build-up of lactic acid in your muscles, which can make them tender or painful.

Constipation and abdominal bloating are very frequent complaints in PMS. Exercise stimulates the smooth muscle of the intestines to contract and relax more efficiently. This in turn prevents or relieves sluggish bowel, constipation, and bloated abdomen caused by impaired bowel function.

There are several reasons why regular aerobic exercise leads to better, more restful sleep. The body has fewer residual chemicals associated with anxiety and tension. The relaxed body state and relative freedom from physical discomfort make it easier to fall asleep and not wake up during the night. As you may already know, relaxing the muscles of the body is an essential part of most relaxation exercises. Regular aerobic exercise preceded by a warmup period and followed by cooling down and stretching does this for your body.

How to and How Much Exercise

The term aerobic refers to the effect that exercise has on your heart and lungs as well as its effect on muscles, bone, connective tissue (ligaments and tendons), and joints. Exercise physiologists have developed optimal heart and respiratory (breathing) rates that help develop the best benefits of exercise without risking damage to your cardiovascular system. But here is the formula you can use right now to calculate your target range. Take the number 220 and subtract your age from it.

For illustration let's say it's 30. Thus 190 beats per minute would be the maximum you should allow during exercise. But you don't need to get your pulse that high. What the experts tell us is that you only need to maintain 65 to 75 percent of your maximum number to produce the desired aerobic benefits. Therefore, since 65 percent of 190 is 123 beats per minute, and 75 percent of 190 is 141 beats per minute, if you can keep your pulse between 123 and 141 beats per minute, you are in what's referred to as your ideal target range. When you do your own calculations, be sure to use your age, not the example.

Your lungs are also involved. Normal resting respirations should increase to 36 to 40 breaths per minutes. Most exercise literature tells beginners to follow this rule: While exercising aerobically, you should have enough breath to talk, but not to sing. Therefore if you're too out of breath to talk, you should slow down, but if you can sing along with your exercise music, you probably need to speed up.

Any responsible authority on exercise will always tell you to see your doctor before starting to determine whether it's safe for you to do regular aerobic exercise. Certainly, we're no exception to this rule. Have a regular checkup, tell your doctor of your plan, and then get set to begin.

When we tell women to exercise, they often ask us what's the best exercise. There isn't one! As long as the exercise gets you into your target pulse and respiration range, it's fine. It is very important to choose exercises you like, or at least, don't hate. Most women like to mix several different types of exercise. That's what we'd recommend.

Begin slowly! Start with fifteen minutes every other day. Gradually increase the time and your level of effort until you reach your goal. That goal should be twenty-five minutes a day, five days a week.

We must stress the need to warm up and cool down. Let's face it, most of us are in a perpetual hurry, and some of us are very competitive. Don't let these tendencies get in your way. In the long run, it just doesn't matter whether you get to your goal in one week or in eight. But people who exercise too long, too hard, and too soon almost invariably hurt themselves and quit or have to stop for a while.

The most common aerobic exercises include: running, jogging, aerobic walking, biking, swimming, stair-climbing, step-aerobics, aerobic dancing, calisthenics, and cross-country skiing.

Be sure to wear the proper clothing when you exercise. The staff in most athletic stores can tell you which foot gear is best for a given sport. It helps to layer your exercise clothing to maintain a comfortable body temperature.

Another essential ingredient to successful and safe exercising is proper hydration and nutrition. It's vital for your health that you consume sufficient water before, during, and after exercising. You can use up more than sixteen ounces of water during twenty-five minutes of aerobic exercise. And you can't rely on feeling thirsty to remind you that you need to replace fluids. By the time you feel thirsty, you may very well be dehydrated. Dehydration can be a serious problem. The best way to prevent it is to drink at least twelve ounces of water before exercise and replace eight ounces every fifteen minutes. You may need even more when exercising in the heat.

Finally, it's important not to become overheated while exercising. Wear a hat to protect your head if you're sensitive to sun. Pour water over your body if you're exercising in the heat. Carry replacement fluids with you. Be very wary of "athletic replacement drinks." In addition to salts and minerals, they often contain sugars that can cause a problem for you.

17

Five Steps to Overcoming the Psychological Problems Associated with PMS

THIS CHAPTER WILL SHOW YOU:

- The importance of listening to your inner voices
- How to identify damaging thoughts
- The most critical step of cognitive restructuring
- How to switch to supportive, encouraging thinking
- The breakthrough technique of re-orienting

As you may have already discovered, having PMS can damage your self-esteem. Being unable to concentrate properly, becoming irritable and unable to function because of seeming depression, can lead to increased negative thoughts and feelings about yourself.

Why not, after all you've encountered? Painful misdiagnoses can often seem like accusations, and the sound of your own thoughts can be depressing.

"I'm still not better after *all these years of therapy* . . ."

"Why do I *always* get so depressed? . . ."

"I must just be a very weak person because I can't seem to do anything right."

If PMS, or other problems in living, have caused you to hear negative nagging thoughts, there are now some very effective ways to deal with these problems. Dr. Martorano's recent book, *Beyond Negative Thinking*, which he wrote with John Kildahl, Ph.D., shows you how to overcome these recurring, damaging thoughts in five easy steps. The process, called "cognitive restructuring," is relatively new and appears to be far more effective than older, traditional analytic methods for getting rid of negative inner dialogues.

Negative thought patterns create a vicious cycle that often continues as "depressogenic" thinking becomes a way of life. Conditioned by your trouble coping with PMS and the enormous stress of the "multiple" roles demanded of today's women, you can easily be led into developing negative thinking about yourself.

The techniques of cognitive restructuring (thought changing) teach you to be assertive in changing the negative recurring thoughts that make your life miserable. Since your style of thinking was learned, it can be unlearned.

A couple of basic concepts are important here. The first is that we experience our thinking as an "inner speech" that we "hear" in the center of our heads. These "spoken" words constitute our thoughts.

The second is that these thoughts can be directly approached and altered to give us a more positive life by using the five-step program below.

Step 1: Listening In

We hear voices (inner speech) in our heads.

These voices need to be monitored (listening in) so that we can connect the negative feelings about ourselves with our recurring patterns of negative thoughts.

For example, you suddenly feel bad because you haven't finished cleaning your house even though you got home late from a tough day at work. You "Listen In" and hear a voice in your head saying, "Irene, you never finish anything." And you start to feel bad.

First, by Listening In you recognize the negative voice. Then, you try to *identify who is actually speaking* and you find that it isn't really your voice but a criticism that your mother (or someone else) used repeatedly to try and get you to finish up your work. The negative thought is actually *her* voice and it is in your head!

What can you do about it?

After correctly identifying any voice in your head other than your own, the first thing you need to do is decide if you really need an "unfriendly" voice in your head. You probably don't! If it is your own unfriendly voice then that's even more important to identify. The world is tough and critical enough for most of us. We don't have to devaluate ourselves.

Unhealthy voices have a tendency to repeat themselves, so that you hear the same negative voice patterns repeatedly triggering off negative mindsets. You may experience these same triggers—the constant self-criticism—year after year, until they are actually programmed in your brain.

Something goes wrong. Instead of trying to solve it, you hear "I'll never get anything right."

Notice the "underlining" because that takes us to the important second step. But remember, Listening In takes practice until you automatically become aware of those negative thoughts.

Step 2: Underline

While you are Listening In, you need to Underline the weakening, damaging words that you experience in your Inner Speech—words like "never" and "anything" in the example above. These damaging words are false generalizations that lead to negative feelings about yourself. (Remember to see if it is someone else in your head who is criticizing you—a critical parent or a difficult teacher or an angry husband just looking to shoot you down.)

The point to remember here is that this is in your head and these negative voices don't belong there.

Underline these words so you can get ready to eliminate them. You already know some of these weakening thoughts and over-generalizations: "Nothing will ever go right." These are what we call the "*tyrannical imperatives*." Hearing over and over in your mind that you should do something or you have to do something. There is often a rigid tyrannical pattern that prevents you from feeling good about yourself. And then this self-demoralization makes you feel even worse.

Here you are premenstrual, your mind not adequately fueled— perhaps because of a lack of progesterone or because you've gone too long without eating—and you are allowing your thoughts to make your life more miserable.

Before, you couldn't confront these voices. But now, armed with the right diagnosis (and starting to feel better as you put your nutritional and medical problems into place), you begin to examine your inner dialogue to connect the negative thought with the bad feeling or the awful behavior.

But what do you do now that you have identified your weakening thoughts? Well, now you put the remarkably effective, easy-to-learn Stopping Technique into effect.

Step 3: Stopping

Stopping is the most critical step of cognitive restructuring. It has been clearly demonstrated that you can actually control exactly what you think and can eliminate negative thought by commanding them to stop. And, even more remarkably, the more strongly you confront these recurring thoughts, the more successful your thinking will emerge.

It's surprisingly easy and effective; you can actually command your thoughts to Stop. All you have to do is to say "STOP" every time you hear a weakening voice in your head.

You don't have to listen to those damaging thoughts. You can crunch them and they will soon disappear entirely from your mind.

Can it really be that simple? No. It isn't quite that simple, but it is that effective. There are a couple of more techniques to learn so that your thoughts will know where to go after you stop the negative ones. After all, you don't want to end up with a blank mind.

After you have stopped the negative thought, you must immediately begin the fourth step to replace the negative thought.

Step 4: Switching

Switching is replacing harmful, negative thinking with good, supportive encouraging thoughts. Stopping and Switching go hand in hand. As soon as you recognize the bad thought (by Listening In and Underlining), intercede directly by Stopping and Switching.

One helpful hint is that it often pays to have in your ready memory a list of five positive thought to switch to. Make the Switching as specific as you can. Don't just say to yourself, "I'll have a better day tomorrow." Try instead, "I'll have a better day tomorrow by starting off with a long invigorating walk and then having a great well-earned breakfast."

Switching can work any situation. Suppose you're sitting in an airplane on the runway, totally panicked that the plane is going to crash. Practice Switching and think ahead to being in your room at the resort, getting ready to go out to that sparkling white beach and into the turquoise water.

Finally there is the fifth breakthrough technique.

Step 5: Re-orienting

In Re-orienting, you take control of your mind by changing the direction of your thinking. This is a much broader technique in which you re-direct yourself to a more satisfying situation.

Let's say you are constantly demoralized in your job. Maybe you can Re-orient your mind. See yourself acquiring new skills and actually visualize yourself in a new more satisfying career. Or even Re-orient your mind to what fun you are going to have at the beach next weekend. It is better to have enjoyable images than critical thoughts. Re-orienting can help you get excited again about your life. Especially if you Re-orient to a totally different and more positive situation.

You can actually now take control of your fully fueled, more alert mind and use this highly successful five-step technique to go in the direction you want.

Remember that earlier voice: "I think of all the years I lost because I didn't know what was wrong with me."

Let's change it right now!

You can hear negative Inner Speech: "Everything I do is . . ." Stop that thought right now and Switch to: "Now I finally recognize what is wrong with me. That's great news. I know how to correct it, and I know I am going to finally feel better. My life is going to be *great.*"

Now, doesn't that feel better?

Interlude

PMS and Your Family

You're probably aware that you're not the only one struggling to cope with your PMS. Your PMS affects your family members as well. Indeed, the longer symptoms have existed without being discussed and dealt with, the greater the amount of damage it effects.

Keeping it all in, or "sparing" family members, simply doesn't work. You may feel that you'll lose control if you tell family members about your problem. Or you may fear that you'll encounter lack of understanding or even criticism. We don't think you should allow those misgivings to curtail openness—clearing up the mystery almost always improves relationships—and when you address this issue openly and appropriately with family members, they can become your allies in coping with it. Our experience has been that the sooner a woman opens up to each member of her family—letting them know what's going on—the sooner the whole family can begin to heal from PMS.

Let's begin with your spouse or mate. Choose a time when you're symptom-free and sit down with him for a discussion. It will help if you let your partner know ahead of time what it is you want to talk about. Come prepared to give him a clear, concise picture of what you've learned from reading this and other literature. You've identified your most troublesome symptoms for yourself; now help your partner to understand the underlying causes behind the way you've been feeling and behaving. Ask your spouse to let you know what he's observed and how it affects him.

You'll undoubtedly be touching upon the sensitive area of the differences in the way you and your partner have perceived particular situations and incidents. As a PMS sufferer, you've never been able to predict accurately when a mood swing or a period of intense irritability would come upon you. You'll need to explain that to your partner because he may have seen you as having more control than you did.

At the same time that you seek and provide understanding, you ought to be aware that your ultimate goal is improvement. PMS can explain what causes of many of the inconsistencies in your life, many of the erratic changes in the way you treat yourself and the people around you, but you should be cautious about allowing it to become an excuse for unacceptable behavior. You're treating your PMS so that you can be happier and make the people you live with happier, too. Your ultimate objective has to be to do away with the out-of-control behavior that's damaging your life.

BEYOND NUTRITION THERAPY

18

Progesterone Therapy

THIS CHAPTER WILL SHOW YOU:

- The background of resistance to natural progesterone therapy
- How progesterone works in the body
- How the right dosage and timing of progesterone is determined
- The evidence for how progesterone works

What do you think would happen if there was an extremely common disease—which ravaged millions of people, destroyed families, and wrecked careers—and suddenly someone found an effective means of treatment that safely eliminated the greatest part of the symptoms?

If you're like most people, you probably imagine that the medical profession would immediately embrace the treatment and nominate its discoverer for a Nobel prize.

It seems to us, too, that that would be the decent and logical thing to do, but, if the disease is Premenstrual Syndrome and the discoverer is Dr. Katharina Dalton, the English clinician we told you about in chapter 1, we know for a fact that the response is different—maybe because it is a woman treating a women's disorder.

In the United States, response to the fact of PMS has been slow, and acceptance of the most effective single therapy for the disorder has been slow and inconsistent.

Dr. Katharina Dalton began treating PMS sufferers in England with natural progesterone in the 1950s. For the past thirty years she and countless other British physicians have been treating significant numbers of women with PMS with natural progesterone and have been achieving excellent results. Progesterone therapy is a noncontroversial and accepted therapy in England. Thirty years of extensive experience has demonstrated *no major side effects* of the therapy. And most other European countries have subsequently embraced natural progesterone therapy, too.

Fortunately, natural progesterone is now widely used in the treatment of PMS. That it isn't universally used may have a lot to do with the peculiarities of the U.S. Food and Drug Administration (FDA).

First, you must understand that progesterone is a *natural* substance. It is derived from wild yams and soybeans, and it cannot be patented by any single drug company. Since the cost of getting FDA approval for a drug in the United States is well over a hundred million dollars, it would take an uncharacteristically altruistic drug company to expend such a sum to take progesterone through all the FDA research requirements for approval, when, at the end of the road, it would have no prospects of obtaining exclusive rights to the drug.

The *FDA Drug Bulletin*, Volume 12, number 1, requires that a drug be labeled, promoted, and advertised only for those uses the safety and effectiveness of which have been established and then approved by the FDA. However the FDA wisely does not limit the manner in which a physician may use an approved drug—that is left to the discretion of the physician. It is understood that unapproved uses may be appropriate and may actually reflect therapies that have been studied and extensively reported in the medical literature. This is, of course, the case with progesterone. The bottom line is that the FDA does not approve or disapprove how a drug is used by a physician in his practice.

This means that while natural progesterone is used for PMS by physicians who understand its therapeutic effectiveness it is not advertised, and therefore, does not become part of the consciousness of most physicians who, once they leave medical school, depend for their further education in what drugs work most effectively for what illnesses on the drug companies and their sales force.

Why Has There Been So Much Trouble Giving Natural Progesterone?

First isolated in 1934, natural progesterone is an odorless white crystalline powder, stable in air and nearly soluble in water. Today it is extracted from yams or soybeans. It is chemically identical to the hormone produced naturally by the human body.

The problem with natural progesterone was deciding how to deliver it. Initially, there was no easily available oral form. The primary routes of administration were rectally and vaginally, using suppositories or a rectal solution. This led to a great variability in absorption as well as terribly poor compliance on the part of patients, since the medication was too inconvenient to take on a regularly scheduled basis. There were, as well, considerable aesthetic and psychological problems using these methods of delivery.

What was really needed was an effective oral form of natural progesterone. The early capsules of oral progesterone produced excessively high blood levels of progesterone with resulting dizziness. A sublingual form was of limited value since it also caused dizziness.

The answer came recently, with the advent of the oral micronized tablets of progesterone in the late 1980s. It is gradually absorbed into the blood stream and represents a dramatic improvement. **Oral micronized progesterone was a giant step forward in the clinical treatment of PMS.**

At the present time, well over 80 percent of our progesterone-receiving patients are treated with this oral preparation. These tablets should be taken with food to decrease the risk of dizziness. Slightly over 15 percent of our patients discontinue the oral micronized form because they feel too drowsy or too dizzy. If this one in six chance occurs, we first decrease the amount administered orally and then, if necessary, add rectal progesterone. If the dizziness persists, we use rectal progesterone alone.

The Functions of Progesterone

The hormone progesterone has a number of very important functions in your body.

- It helps promote the development of the endometrium (lining of the womb).
- It helps maintain pregnancy. In fact, it is frequently used to help women who can't maintain the implementation of the fertilized egg.
- It helps to stabilize glucose tolerance.
- It is important in helping the development of breast tissue.
- It is responsible for the synthesis of corticosteroids in the adrenal cortex.
- It is an immunosupressant—so much so that its relative absence may limit the capacity to respond to allergies and other immune-related disorders.
- It has a known action on the brain that serves as an anticonvulsant, although it is difficult to ascertain whether this is a primary or a secondary action.

Progesterone has a very short half-life in the body, This means it only stays in your body for a limited time. Initially this caused a major limitation in progesterone treatment because when it was given by mouth, it passed via the blood stream to the liver where it was rapidly metabolized. The development of the oral micronized version has a substantially increased length of progesterone's active life in your body, thus extending the therapeutic effects.

This very short half-life really limits any possible negative effects or interactions with other medications, which so far have been minimal.

Progesterone, according to Dr. Dalton, is not carcinogenic. Actually, the reverse seems true and it has been successful used to treat stilbesterol-associated vaginal adenocarcinoma. There are other possible positive implications regarding the use of natural progesterone, such as in post-menopausal hormone replacement therapy. When it is used in conjunction with estrogen, it seems to limit potential difficulties associated with the use of estrogen alone, and recent studies have indicated that progesterone actually helps decrease potential osteoporosis.

WHAT IS THE RIGHT DOSE OF PROGESTERONE?

The dose has to be tailored to the patient, but our usual starting dose of oral micronized progesterone is 300 mgs. of the even-release oral tablet twice a day (morning and night). Some patients need considerably more and some considerably less.

WHAT IS THE PROPER TIMING
FOR PROGESTERONE THERAPY?

Usually, progesterone will start working in one or two days. You should start it at approximately the tenth day of your menstrual cycle. Once it takes effect, you'll start to experience an immediate amelioration of your cognitive symptoms, generally characterized by clearer thinking and a rapid improvement of mood. Relief of swelling and symptoms related to water retention generally takes longer.

You should take progesterone on a daily basis straight through to menstruation. Sometimes it is desirable to increase progesterone administration at a particular time of the month. This increased intervention would most typically be at ovulation or just prior to menstruation.

Fine-Tuning Progesterone Therapy

The two most common clinical errors in progesterone therapy are using an inadequate supply and using the wrong delivery system (such as vaginal suppositories).

If you are currently on progesterone and are not doing well, you should first make sure you are taking natural progesterone and then make sure you are taking either oral micronized or rectal progesterone in adequate amounts.

WHERE CAN I GET NATURAL PROGESTERONE?

Long ago, we made a decision to separate ourselves from any financial gain that could be made from dispensing progesterone. We wanted our patients to receive a clinical decision unrelated to self-interest.

Fortunately, we soon found a dedicated team of pharmacists and support staff at Madison Pharmacy Associates in Wisconsin. Founded in 1982, it is devoted exclusively to helping women with PMS and other hormonal conditions, and we have had great success using their prescription formulations and their support systems. We recommend that you contact them for your progesterone prescriptions. They can be reached by calling 1-800-558-7046 or writing to them at 429 Gawnon Place, Madison, Wisconsin 53719.

WHAT ARE THE MAJOR PROBLEMS ASSOCIATED WITH PROGESTERONE THERAPY?

There are few problems with progesterone therapy, and fewer now than when we started.

As mentioned above, there may be some initial drowsiness or even dizziness associated with the oral form, particularly if it isn't taken with adequate amounts of food. If these side effects persist, we advocate switching to the rectal form.

The principal problem we have found with the rectal form is that it is very poorly absorbed in the swollen bowel, particularly if the patient is constipated. You should take it after a bowel movement. If someone is particularly constipated, we recommend the use of a natural herbal laxative such as Metamucil® to keep the bowel wall clean so that the progesterone will be well absorbed.

The most irritating problem once associated with progesterone therapy was breakthrough vaginal bleeding. It was thought that this was due to progesterone but, actually, it was due to a lack of progesterone while the endometrial lining is reorganizing. Generally speaking, the problem is best solved by increasing, not decreasing, the progesterone.

CAN I BE OVERDOSED WITH PROGESTERONE?

Since progesterone is a natural hormone, the body is well adapted to handling it. Just how excellent that adaptation is can be seen by the fact that during pregnancy, the female body normally handles a progesterone level that is twenty to thirty times higher than the peak levels reached each month during the luteal phase of the menstrual cycle—and it sustains these levels not for two weeks but for nine months. Obviously, therefore, it is very difficult to overdose a woman with progesterone if she has been pregnant. And, in practice, a woman who has never been pregnant can also handle very high levels without complaint.

Is There Any Evidence for How Progesterone Works?

We have come up with dramatic new evidence of the efficacy of progesterone and the way in which it affects patients.

It is crucial to understand that the most important site of action for progesterone is not your reproductive tract but your brain. That's where most PMS symptoms begin, and, with that in mind, you'll have no difficulty understanding why we went where we did for evidence.

We were fortunate enough to have a long-term association with one of the world's foremost neuropsychiatrists, Dr. Turan Itil. His advanced system of computerized electroencephalography has allowed us to utilize technology to demonstrate the remarkable effects of progesterone on the premenstrual brain.

The brain works on electrical currents. You are probably familiar with the term "electroencephalograph" or EEG, as it is commonly abbreviated. The EEG has been used for a long time as a diagnostic tool in clinical psychiatry and neurology. However, its effectiveness was limited because of the necessity to read it visually. Dr. Itil changed all that by applying the computer to read the brain waves. Along the way, he succeeded in accruing a huge data bank of normal values for the different brain waves in the different parts of the brain. Today we are able to put electrodes on a human brain and hook them into our massive computer bank filled with millions of pieces of data and ascertain when a brain is within normal limits.

Using the same system, we can ascertain changes due to the effects of medications on the brain. We have used this technology to observe the effects of progesterone.

We took five women with moderate to severe premenstrual symptoms whose PMS was not wholly alleviated by our full nutritional program and whose profiles met our criteria for progesterone treatment. We did a baseline brainmapping to observe the normal electrical functioning of their brains. Then we gave each woman (none had previously been treated with progesterone) a single 300 mg. tablet of oral micronized progesterone.

The first time we did this even we were amazed at the significant differences in the brain functioning that occurred almost immediately. After a single dose, there were immediate systematic central nervous system effects. These showed great similarity to the results we get with psychoactive drugs that increase alertness, vigilance, and cognition. These results corroborated the verbal reports that we had received from women telling of a "fog" lifting them from their brains.

Such results, statistically verifiable against a huge data base, directly contradict those researchers who state that progesterone has no effect on premenstrual women.

Therefore, if you are having mental symptoms premenstrually that are not significantly alleviated by an appropriate nutritional program, we fully believe that the next logical course of treatment is natural progesterone.

19

The Glucose Tolerance Test: When and What It Means

THIS CHAPTER WILL SHOW YOU:

- What the GTT is like
- What you and your doctor will learn from the GTT
- A review of steps to control your blood sugar level

As we promised in chapter 4, here is a more detailed look at the Glucose Tolerance Test—to give you some sense of what a GTT is like and how you go about interpreting its results.

Each woman who comes to our Center is given a Glucose Tolerance Test as part of her diagnostic workup. The majority of these women will show significant improvement just by going on a diet that excludes most refined carbohydrates, caffeine, and alcohol. The GTT provides us with concrete evidence about for the correlation between PMS and low blood sugar (hypoglycemia). When PMS is the ultimate problem being treated, it is essential to do the test during the premenstrual portion of the month. This is when hypoglycemic effects are most marked. And indeed, many women with PMS will have hypoglycemia only during their premenstruum.

What Will My GTT Be Like?

The GTT is a provocative test, in which you challenge your body with sugar.

You come into the physician's office or laboratory in the morning having eaten and drunk nothing but water for the previous twelve hours. A blood specimen will then be taken to test your fasting blood sugar. A normal fasting level is between 70 to 100 mg%. Then you'll be given a measured glucose solution. In a half hour, the doctor or technician will come back and take another quick blood test and then again half an hour later, and then every hour after that for four or five hours. A lab will then measure the blood sugar levels in each of those specimens and plot a curve showing how your body handles sugar.

You should probably make arrangements to have someone (spouse, relative, neighbor) take you home, because if your hypoglycemia is severe, you may be too confused or tired to return home by yourself safely. You may also want to have some bread and cheese or a glass of milk as soon as possible after the test is completed.

What Will My Physician and I Learn?

You will learn a good deal about whether you have any blood sugar abnormalities, how soon they appear, how severe they are, and how long it is before your blood sugar returns to its baseline.

Normal results (see Figure 5) will be something like the following:

Fasting:	70 to 100 mg%
Peak (30 to 60 minutes):	120 to 160 mg%
Nadir (2 to 4 hours):	60 to 90 mg%

The symptoms that arise during the test and the timing of these symptoms are of considerable diagnostic value. The nadir, or lowest value reached, is obviously of significance and can be a clear indicator of hypoglycemia (see Figure 6), but it is not the only parameter to be considered. A nadir below 60 mg% indicates

Figure 5. Normal Glucose Tolerance Curve

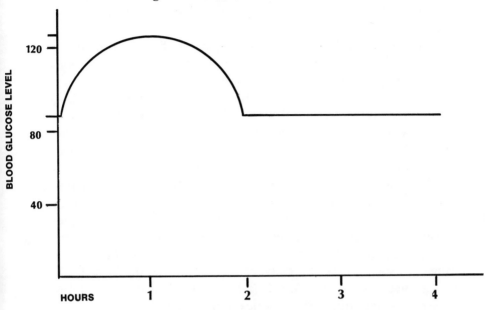

*Figure 6. Typical Hypoglycemic GTT
Curves Associated with 3 or 4 hour "Dips"*

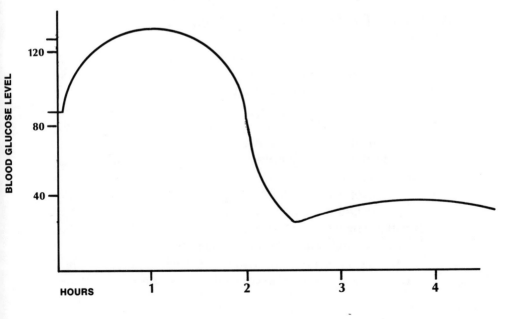

a probable diagnosis of hypoglycemia, but Seale Harris, a noted authority on hypoglycemia, considered that a value below 70 could still support the diagnosis.

Not only are the levels of glucose considered, but also the *rate* at which it falls. A GTT is a dynamic test, and the rate of change is as important as the high and low numbers.

Another factor—used by Dr. Robert Atkins in analyzing GTTs— is what he calls the *delta*. This is the difference between the highest level reached and the lowest. He considers a delta of 100 to be suspicious and a delta of 125 to be a definite indication of blood sugar abnormality.

The symptoms experienced during the GTT are almost as important an indicator as the numbers achieved. Overwhelming weariness, sudden in onset, is a strong indication of a hypoglycemic reaction. In fact, the symptoms of hypoglycemia may be found in a person whose numbers are entirely within the normal range. In such a case, hypoglycemia may still be diagnosed, although less definitively than if it had numerical support. Non-hypoglycemic numbers do not rule out hypoglycemia, they simply fail to substantiate it.

What Do I Do If I Am Hypoglycemic?

If your symptoms and your GTT combine to make it evident that you have some degree of premenstrual hypoglycemia, then take the following steps to prevent a drop in blood sugar level.

- Do not fast or skip meals. Eat three complete meals with three mini-meals in between.
- Eat complex carbohydrates and high-protein foods (see list on page 162.)
- Avoid caffeine and alcohol. These are known to cause a drop in blood sugar level.
- If you are prone to wake up in the morning with a migraine, have a late night snack before going to bed.
- Do not go long intervals without eating, especially when traveling or if you've had a physically strenuous day. Non-

premenstrually your body can go four to five hours without
needing food. Premenstrually, this interval is reduced to two
to three hours.

- If you have an early dinner and afterwards engage in physical activity, be sure to have a high-protein or complex carbohydrate snack afterwards.

A Success Story

Phyllis, a thirty-six-year-old buyer for a retail chain, came to us
from Buffalo. She was having a hard time making it through the
last five days before her period each month. As we reviewed her
general medical history, we learned that she'd been worked up for
narcolepsy (a rare neurological disorder in which a person falls
into a deep sleep without warning). As she described her symptoms, we discovered that her sudden episodes of "falling asleep"
occurred only in the week prior to menses and about one hour after
eating a large meal after skipping a meal. Phyllis noted that she
felt very cold and mentally confused just before she "went out." "I
just can't get myself to drive during that week," she revealed.
"Three times now, I've had to pull off at a rest stop on the Thruway
because I felt it coming on. And once I barely made it!"

We advised Phyllis to have her Glucose Tolerance Test in the
out-patient department of her local hospital. What a response!
Her two-hour blood sugar had plummeted from her baseline of 80
to a dangerous 29. Two months later, Phyllis called to cancel her
second followup appointment. "I'm like a different person," she
exulted. "I must have had this (low blood sugar) for a while now.
My energy's never been better. My briefcase, purse, and coat
pockets are stocked with emergency almonds and dried apricots.
But, you know, since I've begun to eat according to the plan, I need
them less and less. I'm beginning to feel like I can count on myself
again. In fact, I've accepted a promotion and will be traveling
abroad now that I'm feeling well again."

20

Drugs and Their Side Effects

Doctors usually try to help patients suffering from PMS with medications. As you realize by now, a natural solution to Premenstrual Syndrome is almost always better. Even the best of the commonly prescribed medications is usually only temporarily effective.

Nonetheless, I think it's useful for you to have this chapter available for reference. It will help you if your doctor is making a mistake when he prescribes medications for you, and it will also help you if it turns out that some of your symptoms are not simply premenstrual, and your well-informed physician is actually making a good judgment call when he pulls out his prescription pad. In either case, you'll want to know as much as possible about the beneficial effects as well as the undesired side effects of the medication you're being prescribed.

The rest of this chapter will briefly consider the "serious" medications that are most commonly prescribed for women with PMS.

Tranquilizers

Tranquilizers are probably the drugs most commonly prescribed for PMS. They are divided into two major classes: minor and major tranquilizers. The minor tranquilizers are the most familiar and most commonly used. And, of these, the benzodiazepines are the most frequently prescribed.

For patients with anxiety, the benzodiazepines have long been considered the drugs of choice, replacing barbiturates and meprobamate—highly addicting drugs that should not be used for the treatment of anxiety under any circumstances.

The common benzodiazepines include:

Valium® (*diazepam*)
Librium® (*chlordiazepoxide*)
Xanax® (*alprazolam*)
Tranxene® (*chlorazepate*)
Serax® (*oxazepam*)
Centrax® (*prazepam*)
Ativan® (*lorazepam*)

These are relatively safe drugs when used correctly. They have few side effects other than a sedative effect that may impair thinking and motor coordination. That effect is particularly marked if they're used in conjunction with other sedating medications or with alcohol.

However, in spite of their relative safety, they can cause physical dependence. Many patients, particularly those on Xanax®, have to be slowly and carefully withdrawn from their medication. Xanax®, incidentally, was touted as being highly specific for use in PMS, perhaps because it helps alleviate panic attacks. Our experience has been that while it is a highly effective anti-anxiety medication, it loses much of its value because of its potential for abuse.

A relatively new drug, one which does not cause sedation and which has no known potential for abuse and habit formation, is

BuSpar® (*buspirone*). Unfortunately, for most people, it is less effective in reducing anxiety.

If you've been prescribed tranquilizers, you need to ask yourself the following questions:

1. Do they improve or impair my ability to function?
2. Do they sometimes make me drowsy?
3. Can I do my normal tasks? Or do I have to limit myself when I'm taking these medications?
4. Am I starting to build up a tolerance—that is, do I need progressively higher doses to achieve the same effect?
5. Is my doctor carefully monitoring both my dose level and the duration of time I've been on these medications? Keep an exact record of the number of pills you take each day. If you start taking increased amounts, report that to your doctor and ask about it.
6. Am I taking other medications that might increase sedation or side effects? These commonly include: alcohol; anti-histamines and other anti-allergy medications, such as Seldane® or Hismanal®; and Inderal®, a beta blocker that works on the particular receptor sites to limit your anxiety.

   Other possible side effects of drug combinations include visual blurring, ataxia (wobbling), decreased sexual interest, and decreased ability to achieve orgasm. There have been rare reports of aggressive behavior and anterograde amnesia (amnesia with regard to recent experiences). The last problem has, however, been more frequently reported with the use of Halcion®, a sleeping pill.
7. Am I increasing my use of tranquilizers premenstrually? This, of course, brings you back to the question of PMS. If you have it, shouldn't you be looking for better ways to calm yourself down, such as exercising or eating more carefully— especially premenstrually?

The Concept of Half-Life and How It Affects You

Half-life does not refer to the half a life you might be wasting because of PMS but rather to the period of time—after the ingestion of a drug—that is required before the concentration of the drug in your body is decreased by half. Different drugs have different absorption and excretion rates and thus act for different amounts of time on your brain.

Some drugs, such as Ativan® and Centrax®, spend shorter periods of time in your body (have a shorter half-life). Others such as Xanax® and Valium®, have a longer half-life and may even break down (especially true of Valium®) into secondary drugs that will stay in your body for a prolonged period. Generally speaking, we prefer the tranquilizers with a shorter half-life because they don't build up in the body and are less likely to become habit forming.

The Major Tranquilizers

The major tranquilizers are strong drugs that are used mainly to treat psychotic behavior in which the patient is either delusional or hallucinating. If you are placed on such drugs as Thorazine®, Stelazine®, Haldol®, or Navane® and your symptoms only occur premenstrually, your doctor is barking up the wrong tree. Get a consultation immediately as these are dangerous drugs with severe side effects. Their effects can be debilitating or even life threatening.

We do not recommend them for the treatment of PMS, although, in severe postpartum depression, we have sometimes used them with extreme caution for a limited period of time.

The Best Answer

Best with tranquilizers, as with all drugs, is to limit or totally avoid them. If you can treat your premenstrual anxiety successfully with the treatment plan we've outlined in this book, then you won't have to face these drug-related problems.

The Antidepressants

The chapter on depression will help you—with the help of your doctor—to decide whether you need antidepressant medication to deal with a serious level of depression. Here, we'll try to give you the most up-to-date information that we can, but please remember that new and sometimes better drugs are being introduced at a dizzying pace.

The common misconception by patients is that antidepressants are stimulants ("pep pills") that will offer a pick-me-up and relieve fatigue and blues. This simply is not true.

Antidepressants are highly specific medications that are used to treat a very specific disease, commonly called a *biological depression*. Most of these medications act by increasing the levels of certain brain substances (neurotransmitters—usually norepinephrine or serotonin) and thereby improving your mood.

The concept of biological depression has only emerged clearly in recent years with the advancement of brain neuroscience. We are now witnessing the greatest explosion of information regarding the human brain in history. It is almost literally true that each new year doubles or triples the amount of information available. Antidepressants are relatively recent drugs. They were introduced shortly before 1960 and were seldom used before the mid-1970s because therapists were still struggling to solve biological depressions with psychological methods such as analysis. That approach is largely outmoded now. For people who need them, antidepressants are highly specific, truly astonishing drugs, able to transform someone suffering unbearable pain and often stretching out toward suicide in a normal, functioning human being.

If you need antidepressants, you have to work with a doctor with considerable expertise in the field. It will be useful for you to understand the basic types of antidepressants and what their potential for help and harm is.

TRICYCLIC ANTIDEPRESSANTS

The older generation of antidepressants are the tricyclic anti-depressants, and they are found under such names as Elavil®, Tofranil®, Pamelor®, Sinequan®, and Norpramin®.

These can be amazingly effective, but they are very *serious* medications that need to be given correctly. They need to be taken for prolonged periods—usually six months to a year—even after your symptoms have disappeared. Remember also that these drugs need a prolonged time before they start working—usually two to four weeks.

Some side effects of tricyclic antidepressants include: drowsiness, dry throat, low blood pressure (typically producing dizziness if you get up suddenly), sexual dysfunction, and weight gain. Very rarely, these drugs can produce difficulties in the conduction rate of your heart.

SEROTONINERGIC ANTIDEPRESSANTS

The entire field of antidepressants has been revolutionized in the past half-decade by the arrival and use of newer agents with far fewer side effects. These are serotinogenic agents, including the ubiquitous Prozac®, the less well-known Zoloft®, and the brand new Paxil® *(paroxetine)*. These drugs selectively inhibit the uptake of a neurotransmitter, serotonin, which is one of the chief regulators of your mood. A tremendous number of patients who have been depressed their entire lives have suddenly emerged brightly into normal life with the use of these drugs.

These drugs have forced us to reconceive our basic conceptualization of depression. In fact, the effectiveness of these medications has made it clear that the past treatment of depressed patients was really doing a terrible disservice to them. They were treated as people with some inherent psychological weakness, when actually they had a biological deficiency that simply needed to be corrected.

Since Prozac® is the major drug in this area, let us simply mention a few basic facts about it. It usually takes up to three or four weeks to get the maximum effect and should, like other antidepressants, be continued for a minimum of six months. Of course, the period of time will have to be evaluated by both you and your doctor.

There are some side effects including: nervousness, tremulousness (sometimes a hand tremor), headache, nausea, insomnia (or increased vivid dreams), sexual dysfunction—a less frequent symptom—when present, it usually takes the form of anorgasmia (failure to come to orgasm), or akithesia (restless movements).

OTHER GOOD DRUGS

There are a number of other significant, newer antidepressants which are commonly used and which do not yet have a classification by type. These include Desyrel® (*trazodone*) and the newer Wellbutrin® (*bupropion*). Work with your doctor on these. They are highly effective drugs, but they must be taken correctly to get best results and minimize side effects.

MAO INHIBITORS

MAO inhibitors—the common ones include Parnate® (*tranylcypromine*) and Nardil® (*phenelzine*)—*are to be avoided if possible*. They can produce severe and often life-threatening side effects, including large rises in blood pressure especially if taken in conjunction with foods containing tyramine like aged cheeses. Other side effects include: severe, pounding headache; nausea and vomiting; convulsions (seizures); stiff or sore neck; and unusually rapid or pounding heartbeat.

After more than two decades, we seldom, if ever, found them useful. Most patients cannot stay on them for prolonged periods and essentially these are medications *only* for the very, very rare patient who doesn't respond to any other antidepressant.

Nonetheless, over the years, we have seen multitudes of patients who were put on these dangerous drugs. If you are taking an MAO inhibitor or your doctor is suggesting one for you, be extra careful and review all possible choices with him. Needless to say, you should also have made absolutely sure through calendar work and a Glucose Tolerance Test that you are not getting these drugs for PMS. If you have to use them, be sure to secure the help of an expert pharmacologist.

Parlodel®

Prolactin, a hormone that stimulates the secretion of breast milk, can rise greatly if you are under stress or if you have taken certain medications. If its level rises too high, prolactin can lengthen your menstrual cycle and bring on such PMS symptoms as edema and weight gain due to excessive estrogen production. If it were to rise even higher, you might stop menstruating entirely.

There exists a very effective drug called Parlodel® (*bromocriptine mesylate*) that will inhibit the secretion of prolactin from the pituitary. However, this medication has a number of significant side effects including: severe nausea, dizziness, fatigue, headache, and abdominal cramps.

It should not be used as a general-purpose drug against PMS. You should use it only if you have high prolactin levels. To avoid potential side effects start with smaller doses (¼ tablet a day) with evening food and gradually increase doses over a few weeks.

Preparations

A black cloud on the PMS horizon has been the recent introduction of depo preparations of synthetic progesterone as oral contraceptives. Once introduced into your body it will remain active for at least three months.

As you know, the most valuable contribution of the progestogens (synthetic progesterone) is that they inhibit ovulation. However they may have a number of side-effects, the worst of which for you is that they have been shown to lower the plasma concentrations of progesterone, particularly during the luteal (postovulation) phase of the normal menstrual cycle.

This effect has been shown to be dependent upon the dose of the progestogen and can cause a severe, *prolonged intensification of your PMS symptoms*. These progestens can also have other significant side effects, including: breakthrough bleeding, amenorrhea, edema, weight gain, insomnia, somnolence, and blood clots.

As you have learned in the chapter on dysmenorrhea, too many doctors fail to differentiate the various cause of painful menses and have to come to believe that the oral contraceptive (progestogens) that is effective in treating young women with primarily spasmodic dysmenorrhea would also be effective in treating PMS.

It may be up to you to make your physician aware of these differences. It was bad enough to consider that your PMS might be treated with an oral contraceptive, but it is even worse to consider the consequences if this synthetic is stored in your body so that *it may continue lowering your natural body progesterone for several months*.

Medications Are Changing, But Not Necessarily for the Better

Medications may, indeed, be necessary in your life, but as you've read this book, you've probably realized that we think you would be better off without them. The point of this chapter has been to prepare you for the characteristics of drugs that might be prescribed for you as a PMS sufferer. But if you can treat your problem with diet or natural progesterone, or by life-style changes, then we think you'll be a luckier and a happier woman. When your problem is PMS, those therapies will usually do the trick.

21

Treatment-Resistant PMS

THIS CHAPTER WILL SHOW YOU:

- Questions to ask if you don't get better
- The role of the thyroid in PMS
- The six major indicators of yeast infection
- How to distinguish PMS from Chronic Fatigue Syndrome

Many women ask, "But what will I do if I don't get better?" It's a serious question. While most PMS patients improve immediately if given the correct treatment, it's also an unfortunate truth that PMS is like most other medical diseases. A certain percentage of patients just don't get better the first time around. Some of them improve, but not to the degree desirable; an even smaller percentage fail to respond to treatment at all.

In such treatment-resistant cases, the understanding and cooperation of the patient is often as important as the expertise and experience of the physician. We assume that if you're even reading this chapter it's because your treatment isn't going as smoothly as you would like. So let's go through a series of questions and decisions that should ultimately make it clear why you aren't getting better.

Are You Getting the Right Treatment for PMS?

As you've learned, PMS treatment breaks down into two parts: nutritional therapy and progesterone therapy.

If you are under thirty without a history of multiple pregnancies, and prolonged use of the pill, it is probable that you'll experience considerable relief from your symptoms if you apply the nutritional program outlined in this book.

If your symptoms persist is spite of this program, then you have to look closely to see whether you are really following all the different aspects of the program.

KEEP A FOOD JOURNAL

Your food journal should be a meticulously maintained document. Recording the exact times, the exact foods and quantities of foods eaten, and the exact symptoms and the time of their onset is absolutely essential. Having this information can protect you from two common and catastrophic errors: falling prey to the food gap and making food mistakes.

It is extremely important—especially if you are busy and active— to remember the recommendation of frequent, small meals. Going more than three hours without eating can cause you blood sugar to drop. Once it has fallen, it is much harder to get it back up to normal, and you may be confronted by sugar cravings so intense that they become irresistable, leading to bingeing and bad results.

Be sure you are choosing the right foods. Don't believe that the word "health" on a food package means that it's healthy for you. That healthy bran muffin may be loaded with corn syrup. Anything that has flour in it most likely has some form of sugar in it, too.

Avoid fruit juices entirely and be careful of citrus fruits, especially on an empty stomach. Avoid fruits like raisins and grapes that are high in natural sugar. They simply aren't good for your metabolism. Their "natural" sugar gets translated into an immediate rise in blood sugar followed by the inevitable devastating drop.

Beware of So-Called Sugar-Free Foods

When Cheryl, visiting nurse of forty-two, came to us, she had many troubling symptoms. These included bloating, breast tenderness, right-sided headaches, sudden fatigue, angry outbursts, and mood swings. Her GTT showed that her three-hour sugar level dropped to 55, and had not returned to her baseline of 70 by the end of the fifth hour. We counseled her on diet, nutritional supplements, and aerobic exercise.

Three months later she'd gotten relief from all her fluid retention symptoms, but her low blood sugar symptoms would crop up for two or three days each month. Puzzled, we had our nutritionist meet privately with Cheryl to assess her diet. At first it seemed right on target. Denise, our nutritionist, spotted the culprit right away. Cheryl kept stopping at a "health food" store to buy "natural, sugar-free" muffins after seeing one of her patients. These natural, sugar-free muffins turned out to be loaded with concentrated fruit juice. After eliminating them from her diet, those troubling and persistent blood sugar symptoms disappeared.

If you have low blood sugar symptoms, you can avoid Cheryl's experience by purchasing only foods that list ingredients. Words like "natural" and "sugar-free" can be misleading, and often refer only to refined sugar. When you've gotten complete relief of symptoms through at least three consecutive cycles, you can begin to reintoduce items like Cheryl's muffins one at a time. This way you can assess whether or not you can tolerate them.

When you look at your food journal try to notice the patterns that will explain the relation between what and when you're eating and the timing of your symptoms. Eventually, you may be able to identify correlations between specific, bad reactions and certain foods ingested hours earlier. The symptoms may not even occur until the next day.

What we call the *"Lag Phenomenon"* is not uncommon. Your own particular metabolism will determine how long the lag is between a certain nutritional error and the appearance of symptoms. The food journal is something you should keep in order to learn about your own body.

Are You Using Progesterone Correctly?

If a carefully planned program of nutritional improvement does not result in a sufficient alleviation of your symptoms, then you will presumably have gone on to use natural progesterone. Here, too, there is room for error.

If you have all the signs of PMS, and you're on progesterone, and you fail to respond, several questions need to be asked.

1. Are you sure you're getting the right form of progesterone—natural progesterone, not synthetic?
2. If you're taking an oral preparation of natural progesterone, are you sure it is the *micronized* form, which is more effectively absorbed?
3. Are you taking enough? Be sure to check the dosage with your doctor. Generally speaking an oral dose of 300 mgs. twice a day (with meals) is an average effective dose.
4. Ask your doctor if you should replace or supplement the oral form with a *rectal solution*, or some other form of delivery. Some patients simply do not respond to one or the other form of progesterone and need a different delivery system. (Our experience has been that oral micronized progesterone works in approximately 80 percent of all cases. Usually, if the oral progesterone doesn't totally suffice, we *add* a rectal solution of progesterone. We prefer the *solution* to the suppository because of better absorption.)
5. If the rectal solution does not seem to be working, then ask yourself a further question: Are you chronically constipated? A significant number of women with PMS are constipated because the bowel wall becomes swollen due to retained fluid (edematous) in the premenstrual phase. In

order for rectal progesterone to be effectively absorbed, it is necessary to have a clean surface area. If you're not responding, and you're constipated, consider the daily use of a mild herbal laxative in the premenstrual phase of your cycle to clean the bowel and facilitate absorption of progesterone. To check your absorption, look and see if almost all of the white chalky material is being passed out in your stool. If it is, then you're not absorbing it correctly.

Three Other Problems

You need to consider the possibility that you may be suffering from more than one problem. As you know, having PMS doesn't exclude your having other disorders. *Mental disorders* may play a role.

You should also be sure to have a thorough physical exam with laboratory studies. There are three major disorders that need to be dealt with in detail and that may explain the persistence of problems even after you've had the appropriate treatment for your PMS. They are thyroid disease, yeast infections, and Chronic Fatigue Syndrome (CPS).

The Role of the Thyroid in PMS

Consider the following symptoms of an underactive thyroid gland: weight gain, painful joints, tearfulness, mood swings, fatigue, and irritability. Almost sounds like PMS, doesn't it?

It is known that the thyroid gland is involved in stimulating the hypothalmus of the brain, which then causes the pituitary gland to release FSH and LH (follicle-stimulating hormone and lutenizing hormone)—the initiators of the menstrual cycle. A pivotal article, by Dr. R. L. Reid and Dr. S. S. Yen in 1981, suggested that PMS would result from changes in this system.

Simply put, if the thyroid gland is underactive and brain hormones aren't released, then your progesterone production may be diminished to the point where you have PMS. And you might not get better until some form of thyroid medication is added to your regimen to help restore progesterone production. Take the following test to help you see if an underactive thyroid may be limiting your improvement.

Please answer each question on a *0 to 10 scale* (10 being most severe) and note if the symptoms occur all month long or only premenstrually.

Symptoms	Number rating	All month	Pre-menstrually only
Do you feel cold frequently?			
Are you excessively weak?			
Is your skin dry?			
Do you tire excessively?			
Is your speech slow?			
Is your sweating decreased?			
Is your skin cold?			
Does your tongue often feel thick?			
Does your face swell?			
Is your hair getting coarser?			
Is your skin excessively pale?			
Is your memory often impaired?			
Are you constipated frequently?			
Have you experienced weight gain beyond ordinary expectations?			
Have you experienced recent hair loss?			
TOTAL:			

If your ratings total more than 75, you may have a thyroid problem. If your total is more than 100, it is more likely that your thyroid is involved.

WHAT IF YOUR DOCTOR TESTED FOR THYROID DEFICIENCY AND FOUND YOU NORMAL?

All too often we hear women say, "I couldn't have any thyroid problems because my doctor tested it and . . ."

That may be exactly what happened to you. Unfortunately, experienced clinicians have long found the normal range of thyroid blood tests to be far less sensitive than they would wish. Over the years, we at PMS Medical have seen countless women with laboratory tests (for thyroid) within normal limits who clearly presented a clinical picture of a mild low-grade hypothyroidism.

If you did the thyroid checklist above, and your symptom ratings totalled 75 to 100, we recommend you take your temperature when you first wake up in the morning. If done orally, this should be for a minimum of five minutes *before* you get out of bed in the morning.

If the temperature is consistently one degree or more lower than normal (98.6° F.), we would consider adding thyroid supplements on a trial basis. Usually treatment consist of thyroxine replacement, generally in the form of low doses of Synthroid® (*levothyroxine sodium*) or Cytomel® (*liothyronine sodium*). Although in the normal course of treatment such replacement therapy is usually given after progesterone has failed to alleviate all symptoms, we have found that in some cases where thyroid is given first, it alone may suffice to trigger the brain's neuroendocrine system into proper functioning.

One type of patient that we have found unusually responsive to thyroid medication is a woman who complains of frequent chills and diminished sexual desire. These complaints, coupled with PMS symptoms and often found in somewhat older women, can frequently be a clue for thyroid deficiency.

If you have not responded to your PMS treatment course, it is essential that you consider thyroid dysfunction. If you choose a thyroid trial, work closely with your doctor to make sure your thyroid dose level is correct. If it's too high, you may experience nervousness, tremulousness, and insomnia. If it is too low, you may not reach a thyroid blood level sufficient to retrigger your neuroendocrine system into functioning again.

Yeast Infections

No discussion of unresponsive PMS would be complete without some mention of yeast infections and their role in intensifying PMS.

Doctors (and patients, too) are becoming more and more aware that chronic overgrowth of *Candida albicans* yeast can present a complex problem of diagnosis and treatment. *Candida* is one of the more than 400 species of indigenous flora (bacterias and yeasts) resident in the human intestinal tract. During periods of stress, or as the result of an impaired immune responsee, *Candida* can proliferate. In its invasive fungal state, it produces *rhizoids*, which, with their very long rootlike structures, can penetrate the mucous membrane in the intestine or the vagina. This results in symptoms such as fatigue, depression, inability to concentrate, headaches, sinusitis, bloating, food sensitivities, and mouth infections (thrush).

Women appear to be far more susceptible to this infestation, partially as the result of hormonal changes that can affect the growth of yeast. Since the yeast is a normal part of your body, there is no specific laboratory test that can detect its overgrown form.

If you have the above symptoms and are not getting better, it is crucial that you carefully develop your own history and present it to a physician familiar with yeast infections.

SIX MAJOR CLUES

These are the important clues for diagnosing a yeast infection:

1. *Do you have a history of prolonged antibiotic use?* Long-term antibiotic use can destroy some of the other bacteria in the intestine and vagina that tend to compete with and discourage the overgrowth of *Candida*.
2. *Have you used oral contraceptives recently?* They can cause changes in the vaginal membrane that allow yeasts to multiply more rapidly. It's estimated that up to 35 percent of women on the Pill have yeast infections.
3. *Have you used steroids such as cortisone or prednisone recently?* Steroids suppress the immune response and pave the way for yeast infections.
4. *Is you diet rich in sugars or starch foods?* These can cause *Candida albicans* to multiply more rapidly as yeast feeds on sugar.
5. *Do you frequently eat foods with a high yeast or mold content?* Foods such as cheese, mushrooms, alcohol, and most breads and pastries encourage the multiplication of yeast.
6. *Have you had multiple pregnancies?* The fluctuating hormone levels of pregnancy appear to make women more susceptible to yeast infection.

When it appears that a woman has the symptoms of *Candida albicans*, we check for recurrent vaginitis (cultures often help) and on physical examination we look for recurrent white spots on the throat. A treatment plan usually involves dietary changes with an emphasis on consuming lots of vegetables and high protein foods such as fish, eggs, and nuts.

For women who do not respond to dietary changes alone, we frequently recommend a prolonged course of drugs such as Nystatin®, which kills yeast and yeastlike fungi.

Fatigue and PMS

One of the most difficult premenstrual symptoms to treat is fatigue, principally because so many different factors can cause it. Yeast infections and thyroid disorders are major contributors, and so is the newly defined disorder Chronic Fatigue Syndrome (CFS).

CFS is hard to delineate medically because the highly subjective nature of the complaints cover a wide range of symptoms, including not only fatigue but also joint pain, impaired thinking, memory loss, and depression. The real cause of CFS is not clear, but certainly many of its sufferers have been shown to have CEBV— Chronic Epstein-Barr Virus—first identified in 1964. Epstein-Barr is very widespread, and it strikes women three times as often as men, possibly because of some innate difference between the male and female immune systems.

CEBV has a very insidious onset, and its duration may vary from weeks to years. It usually strikes people between the ages of twenty-five and forty-five, and it appears to affect a preponderance of white, upper middle-class professionals.

It is often very hard to distinguish between PMS and CEBV because there is so much symptom overlap, and therefore it is very important to observe the *postmenstrual* period to see if there is a substantial alleviation of the fatigue. That would, of course, point to PMS. On the other hand, if the symptoms have a more sudden onset, almost like an attack, that would indicate a more likely diagnosis of CEBV. However, since both disorders are common, it is far from rare for them to coexist in the same person. In that case we follow PMS treatment with medical treatment for CEBV when necessary.

It is best to proceed this way and to follow up PMS treatment with a re-evaluation of the entire clinical picture because the blood tests for Epstein-Barr remain crude and inaccurate—up to 30 percent of those suffering the disorder may have CEBV antibody levels within the normal range. Conversely, there are people who show high Epstein-Barr antibody levels without significant symptoms.

Treatment-Resistant PMS and You

Since PMS *should* respond to an effective treatment plan such as the one explained in this book, one *does* have to look carefully when that result does not occur. Our experience has been that generally the lack of response is caused by other disorders like the ones described in this chapter. In such a difficult situation, it's important for you to be *determined* enough to ferret out those other disorders.

22

How to Find the Best Help for Your PMS

THIS CHAPTER WILL SHOW YOU:

- What to ask yourself about your doctor
- What to ask your doctor
- What to do if your doctor doesn't measure up
- That YOU are the best source of help in conquering your PMS

If you're reading this book, you've probably already located the best source for your PMS—YOU! This book is designed to be your treatment partner. Don't just read it and throw it away: underline and outline what pertains to you. If you keep in mind exactly what you need to do—and your PMS is of moderate dimensions—it's likely that you'll be able to control your symptoms effectively.

For those readers whose symptoms are not immediately responsive to nutritional intervention, there is a well-developed network of help throughout the nation. First, however you might consider investigating your relationships with your physicians to see if it's possible to have one of them for a treatment partner.

Take a look at our simple two-part system.

The First Part: Questions to Ask Yourself

1. *Does the doctor have enough time for me?* Treating PMS takes time, and a doctor who was truly wonderful in delivering your children or treating your flu may still be too overwhelmed by other needs to give you and your PMS the time it requires.

   There's no need to disrupt your relationship. Simply use this doctor for what he or she is best qualified to treat.

2. *How has this doctor responded to questions I've asked in the past?* Does the doctor really *listen* to you or just breeze past on the way to the prescription pad? If your doctor simply zooms by, pin him or her down or find a new treatment partner.

3. *Is the doctor willing to accept me as an active partner?* Almost invariably, treatment results improve dramatically when a patient does her homework. Keeping careful records, charting symptoms, noting results as carefully as possible—all these really count. This question has a lot to do with questions 1 and 2. If you do your share of homework, is the doctor going to have the interest and the time to utilize your efforts to help you get better? You certainly don't want the doctor to make decisions for you without considering the information you've gathered, without any interaction.

The Second Part: Questions to Ask Yourself

It's only in the past decade that women have started to effectively query their doctors. We believe it is an important part of the treatment process.

Try to remember that *you are employing your doctor*. Cooperation and mutual respect are the keys. In order to know whether you've come to the right doctor, you'll need to know what your doctor knows about PMS and that means asking him certain critical questions.

1. *Does the doctor accept PMS as a discrete medical entity and not a psychological weakness in women?*

    Unless the answer is an unequivocal yes, you're almost certainly sitting in the wrong examination room.

2. *Ask how he or she proposes to treat PMS.*

    If the doctor approaches your problem with a quick fix prescription pad or thinks a modest dose of vitamin B_6 is the entire answer, you're probably going to need assistance. If the treatment plan doesn't bear many similarities to the one we've explained in this book, then the doctor is not well informed in the area.

3. *Does the doctor believe in hypoglycemia? Does he or she have an adequate grasp of the significance of nutritional corrections in treating PMS?*

    Your partner in treating PMS simply must have some grasp of the nutritional basics. If your doctor knows nothing about the foods you should avoid, or scoffs at Glucose Tolerance Tests, then why are you coming to this person for advice?

4. *Is the doctor willing to learn?*

    Assuming the doctor knows something about PMS and its treatments, is he or she willing to absorb and accept more information from you? If you present what you've learned in this book in a non-threatening manner, is he or she willing to listen? You're responsible for presenting that information in a reasonable, friendly, non-shaming way. No doctor can know everything; there's far too much to know. But if you suggest important points in your treatment plan, and your doctor doesn't seem interested in considering them, you may have the wrong doctor. Of particular importance is willingness to give you a Glucose Tolerance Test premenstrually when your symptoms are at their worst. **Make sure the doctor is aware of the specific timing of the test.**

An Early Warning System
for Evaluating Your Physician

Be wary if:

1. Your doctor doesn't know the difference between synthetic progestogens and natural progesterone. If he or
   she seems to be referring to them interchangeably, that's
   a bad sign.
2. Your doctor dismisses the symptoms of low blood sugar
   or scoffs at the concept of hypoglycemia.
3. Your doctor immediately resorts to the prescription pad.
   Trying to tranquilize you without first establishing the
   cause of your symptoms is a poor approach.
4. Oral contraceptives are prescribed for PMS. These are
   synthetic forms of progesterone.

If your doctor measures up to the standard set by these leading
questions, then you are probably in good hands, and you should
employ him or her as your partner in treating PMS.

Even if your doctor turns out to be an entirely adequate partner, he or she may still not be able to work out an entire PMS diet
for you. So use the information in this book. If you have any
questions about nutrition ask your doctor or seek the help of a
qualified nutritionist. You might even want to save some money by
going to your local library and reading up on any highly specific
nutritional problems you're experiencing.

You'll notice we're still placing the major responsibility on your
shoulders. After all, you're the one who's suffering.

What If the Doctor Doesn't Meet My Criteria?

If your doctor doesn't measure up, the solution depends upon
where you live. If you live in an isolated rural area, your choices

may be very limited, and you may have to do much of the work yourself. For additional access, you can call the national network of PMS Access at 1-800-222-4767. The people at the network are very helpful and friendly and will probably be able to provide you with a long listing of the nearest competent PMS specialists. They'll also answer questions about PMS, suggest books you can read, and recommend other organizations you can talk with.

Now that you've read this book, we hope you'll agree that not only can PMS have a tremendous impact in many areas of your life, but identifying it—and not being fooled by it—requires a searching analysis of the things that ail you. To some extent, medicine still hasn't caught up to the reality of PMS. Therefore, in this area YOU must be the master architect of your blueprint to reclaim health.

A careful evaluation of your symptoms—with the aid of your menstrual calendar—will make it possible for you to have a very good idea of what symptoms PMS is responsible for even before you consult a physician.

You'll be able to identify and strip away your PMS masks. They may be as simple as headaches and irritability. Or they may extend into many of the wide range of less obvious symptoms that we discussed in Part II of this book. Depression, panic attacks, chronic fatigue, dysfunctional behavior related to alcohol, and many, many other types of mental and physical masks can all be traced to the hormonal disturbances in your menstrual cycle.

Many women get a dramatic emotional lift from learning they have PMS. Just the knowledge that their suffering isn't mental illness or some dread disease changes their evaluation of themselves and the world around them. Equally important is finding out what ailments are not related to PMS. At least that knowledge is a step in the direction of finding out the true cause.

We won't say too much more here about misdiagnosis and mistreatment. The book has been devoted to giving you the knowledge to protect yourself against these assaults. Now you know just how common it is to be treated for years with therapies that seem superficially well-suited to handling your symptoms (if it were not that your symptoms are really the result of PMS). And, you certainly have learned that, when you have PMS, it's the PMS that must be treated and not the symptoms.

We've shown you how easy it is to treat PMS once it's been identified. PMS is *not* one of the world's more difficult disorders to manage—it's simply one of the world's most widespread and most misidentified syndromes. The PMS patient who does not show improvement once she goes on an appropriate nutritional plan is rare, and the woman who does not get substantially better after the correct administration of natural progesterone is even rarer.

Now you have the information necessary to launch a full-scale assault on Premenstrual Syndrome. Most of you will find that if you strictly follow the recommendations we have given you, success will come almost as a matter of course. Some of you will have a slightly harder and more complicated path to wellness. But PMS is conquerable. Your own commitment and the choice of a knowledgeable and responsive physician will eventually free you of a burden that you've done nothing to deserve.

Index

abortion, 36, 43
adrenalin, 55, 98
Advil®, 129, 130
alcohol, 31, 36, 87, 102, 103, 115, 119–126, 169–170, 201; and low blood sugar, 123–124, 162; and tranquilizers, 209; and women, 121–123
allergic responses, 48, 85
American Journal of Clinical Nutrition, The, 171
American Psychiatric Association, 82
Anacin®, 94
Anaprox®, 94
anorexia nervosa, 49
anxiety, 20, 37, 48, 89–95; definition of, 89–90; results of, 91; self-diagnosis test for, 92
arthritis, 93; rheumatoid, 46–47
asthma, 47, 48
Ativan®, 62, 103, 139, 208,210
Atkins, Dr. Robert, 204

Basal Body Temperature (BBT), 157–158
Berchtold, Nancy, 140
Biphasal Hormone Replacement Therapy (BHRT), 142–145
bloating, 33, 36, 37, 42, 48, 49, 147–149, 163–164
blood sugar. *See* glucose; hypoglycemia
brain functioning, 51–52, 85–86
brain mapping, 26, 144–145, 199–200
brain tumors, 21, 112
breast feeding, 139

British Migraine Association, 110
bronchitis, 47
bulimia, 49
BuSpar®, 104, 208–209

caffeine, 62, 93–94, 162, 169–170, 201
calcium, 171–172. *See* also minerals
carbohydrates, 54, 57, 100, 162, 201; complex, 161, 162; healthy snacks, 163; list of foods rich in complex, 162; simple versus complex, 54
CAT scans, 21, 111–112
Centrax®, 139, 208, 210
Chronic Epstein-Barr Virus (CEBV), 226
Chronic Fatigue Syndrome (CFS), 47, 226
cognitive restructuring, 154, 183–188
colitis, ulcerative, 47
contraceptives, oral, 42, 87, 129
cravings, food, 36, 52, 56, 124; and compulsive eating, 49. *See* also eating habits
Cytomel®, 223

Dalton, Katharina, 14–15, 24–25, 43, 136, 193, 194, 196
Depakote®, 82
depression, 20, 36, 37, 42, 45, 46, 47, 48, 52, 65–79, 93, 211; types of, 73. *See* also manic depression; postpartum depression
Depression After Delivery, 140
Desyrel®, 213
Dexatrim®, 93

disorders, psychological, 14, 221
diuretics, 31, 93, 148. *See also*
　bloating; weight gain
dysmenorrhea, 42, 43, 93, 129–133;
　congestive, 131; self-test diagnosis
　for, 130; spasmodic, 129–130.
　See also endometriosis

eating habits, 36, 58, 61; restructuring
　to combat PMS, 153, 159, 161–163,
　175, 218; sample recommended
　meal plan, 174–175. *See also*
　cravings, food; nutrition
Elavil®, 46, 65, 67, 212
endometriosis, 131–132. *See also*
　dysmennorhea
estrogen, 40, 41, 42, 51, 112, 147
Evening Primrose Oil, 149, 173–174, 175
Excedrin®, 93
exercise, 62, 154, 155–156; as therapy,
　177–181

fatigue, 45–46, 47, 52, 93; and PMS,
　226; combatting, 154
FDA Drug Bulletin, 194
feedback loop, 51
feminists, 25, 84
fibroids, 132
Fiorinal®, 111
fluid retention, 147–149, 163–164. *See
　also* bloating; diuretics; weight gain
Follicle Stimulating Hormone (FSH),
　40, 41, 221
Food Journal, 114, 116, 159–160, 218–
　220; Lag Phenomenon with, 220
Frank, Dr. Robert T., 24
Freud, Sigmund: legacy of, 13, 19–20
fructose, 58. *See also* glucose; hypo-
　glycemia

Gatorade®, 59
glaucoma, 47
glucose, 24, 51–52, 53–60, 100, 113,
　144–145; and alcohol, 123–124

glucose tolerance, 24
Glucose Tolerance Test (GTT), 59–60,
　74, 76, 84, 87, 98, 106, 201–205,
　214; description of, 202; function
　of, 202–204. *See also* hypoglycemia
Greene, Dr. Raymond, 25

Halcion®, 209
Haldol®, 104, 139, 210
Harris, Dr. Seale, 24, 204
headaches, 28, 42, 93, 107–118; and
　food, 114–115; definitions of, 108–
　109; migraines, 46, 49, 55, 93, 164;
　related to PMS, 110–114, 116–118;
　related to tension, 108
heart problems, 97–106; murmur, 21;
　palpitations, 29, 55. *See also* mitral
　valve prolapse
Hismanal®, 209
hormones, 40, 44, 51; and menopause,
　142–145; balance of, 40–41, 43, 86,
　136, 142–145; counterregulatory,
　55. *See also* adrenalin; estrogen;
　Follicle Stimulating Hormone;
　insulin; Luteinizing Hormone;
　progesterone; prolactin
Hydrodiuril®, 31
hyperthyroidism, 47, 221–224; self-
　diagnosis test for, 222; treatment
　for, 223–224
hypoglycemia, 48, 49, 52, 53–55, 56–
　59, 71–72, 73–74, 85–86, 113, 121,
　123–124, 160–161, 201; diagnosis
　from GTT, 202–204; forms of, 73;
　treatment of, 161–163, 204–205. *See
　also* glucose; Glucose Tolerance Test
hysterectomy, 36, 43, 44, 45

immune system, 47, 48
Inderal®, 111–112, 209
insulin, 54–55
irritability, 28, 30, 36, 37, 48, 52, 55,
　93. *See also* anxiety; tension
Itil, Dr. Turan, 199–200

Johns Hopkins Medical School, 122

lethargy, 47, 48
Librium®, 208
lithium, 82, 83–84
Luteinizing Hormone (LH), 40, 41, 221

MacKinnon, Drs., 52
Madison Pharmacy Associates,
    173, 198
magnesium, 93, 171–172
manic depression, 81–88; self-
    diagnosis test for, 83
Martorano, Dr. Joseph, 15, 138
medical establishment: American, 13,
    14, 24, 25, 66; American physicians'
    view of women, 23, 99–100;
    British, 25
Mellaril®, 104
memory lapses, 52, 93, 126, 141
menopause, 141–145
menstrual calendar, 32–35, 46, 214;
    and depression, 74–79; and mood
    swings, 86–87; record-keeping,
    153, 155
menstrual cramps, 28, 42
menstrual cycle: review of hormonal
    activity during, 40–41, 112–113
menstruation, 36
Metamucil®, 198
Midol®, 94
minerals, 171–172, 175. *See also*
    calcium; magnesium; potassium
miscarriage, 36, 43
mitral valve prolapse, 21, 97, 102–105.
    See also heart problems
mood swings, 29, 74–75, 81–88
Morgan, Maureen, 15
Motrin®, 129, 130
MRIs, 21, 111–112

Nardil®, 69, 104, 213
Navane®, 210
New York Center for Brain Study, 144

NoDoz®, 93
Norpramin®, 212
nutrition, 23, 31, 55, 56–59, 72, 86, 87,
    105; recommendations to improve,
    153, 155–156, 161–176
Nystatin®, 225

obsessive compulsive behavior, 48
Okey, Dr. R., 24
ovarian cysts, 132
ovulation, 41; determination of onset,
    157–158

Pace, Dr. Nicholas, 124
Pamelor®, 212
panic attacks, 29, 37, 55, 97–106;
    definition of, 98; self-diagnosis
    test for, 99
parasites, intestinal, 47, 85
Parnate®, 104, 213
Parlodel®, 214
Paxil®, 212
Percocet®, 111
peptic ulcer, 47
PMS. *See* Premenstrual Syndrome
PMS Access, 233
PMS depression, 65–79. *See also*
    depression
PMS Medical, 15, 20, 144, 223
Ponstel®, 129, 130
postpartum depression, 43, 68, 90,
    135–140, 210
potassium, 31, 93, 148, 165, 171–172
pregnancy, 36, 42
Premarin®, 143
Premenstrual Syndrome: average age
    at onset, 45; definition of, 35; defini-
    tion of treatment, 218; development
    of, 30; diagnosis of, 20–21; differen-
    tial diagnosis for, 39–40, 46–50, 82,
    91; discussing at home, 189–190; dis-
    cussing with a physician, 229–232;
    doctors' lack of understanding of,
    19, 20–23, 73–74, 194–195; effects

on family, 189–190; history of, 24–
26; masks of, 13, 14, 19, 20, 35; misdiagnosis of, 20–23, 32, 35, 46;
misdiagnosis of, as anxiety, 89–91;
misdiagnosis of, as depression, 65–
79; misdiagnosis of, as heart problems, 102–105; misdiagnosis of, as
manic depression, 82–86; misdiagnosis of, as migraines, 107–114;
misdiagnosis of, as panic attacks,
97–102; mistreatment of, 13, 19,
20–21; politics of, 25; precipitating
factors of, 42–45, 55; relation to
menstrual cycle, 14, 25, 26, 30, 35,
49–50; self-diagnosis of, 32–38; statistics of, 19; symptom recognition,
20; symptoms of, 19; symptoms, list
of, 27–29; symptoms, psychological, 20, 52, 91; treatment-resistent,
217–227
prescription drugs, 15, 87, 88, 207–
215; and the menstrual cycle,
69–70; antidepressants, 69, 70, 71,
72, 101, 211–214; antidepressants,
serotoninergic, 212–213; antidepressants, tricyclic, 103, 212;
antihistamines, 103, 209; barbituates, 104, 208; benzodiazines,
103, 208–209; MAO inhibitors, 69,
213–214; tranquilizers, 62, 72, 95,
208–211
Procycle®, 173
Prozac®, 69, 86
productivity: decline in, 36; rescheduling activities to improve,
153, 155
progesterone, 15, 40, 41, 42, 45, 51,
55–56, 84, 112, 136, 138, 149, 160;
availability of natural forms of, 198;
depo-preparations of synthetic
form of, 214–215; development of
natural forms of, 195; efficacy of
natural forms of, 199–200; functions of natural forms of, 196;

production in the body at ovulation, 157; medicinal doses of natural form of, 195–196, 197, 199;
natural forms of, 23, 32, 114, 118;
PMS therapy with natural form of,
193–200, 220–221; relation to
sodium, 163–164; resistance in U.S.
to natural forms of, 193–196; side
effects of natural, 198–199; synthetic forms of, 23, 32, 42, 143–145;
uses of natural form of, 196–197
prolactin, 136; inhibitting production
of, 214
protein, 100; foods high in, 161, 162
Provera®, 31–32
Prozac®, 212–213

Rapid Cycling Disorder, 82
Rcid, Dr. R. L., 221
relaxation exercises, 62, 154
Robb, Dr. E. L., 24

salt. *See* sodium
Seldane®, 209
Serax®, 62, 208
Sinequan®, 212
sleep, 61–62, 86, 139
sodium, 160, 165; and PMS, 163; foods
high in (to avoid), 167–168; foods
low in, 165–167; hints to reduce,
164–165
Southern Medical Journal, 24
spironolactone, 148
Stelazine®, 104, 210
stress, 36, 113; rescheduling activities
to reduce, 153, 155
Stress Journal, 114, 116
Sudafed®, 117
sugar, 31; hidden, in processed and
"natural" foods, 175, 219. *See also*
glucose and fructose
suicide and suicidal thoughts, 52,
66–67, 70, 84, 121, 137–138
Synthroid®, 223

Tegretol®, 67, 69
tension, 48, 89–95; definition of, 90; results of, 91; self-diagnosis test for, 92
Thorazine®, 104, 210
thyroid. *See* hyperthyroidism
Tofranil®, 67, 69, 101, 211
Tranxene®, 208
tubal ligation, 36, 43, 45, 120

United States Food and Drug Administration (FDA), 194

Valium®, 103, 208, 210
vitamin A, 169, 170, 171, 172
vitamin B Complex, 86, 169, 172
vitamin B$_6$, 31, 84, 86, 169, 170, 173
vitamin C, 85, 169, 173
vitamin therapy, 15, 93, 155, 175; recommended daily amounts, 172–173

water retention, 48. *See* sodium
Wellbutrin®, 213
weight gain, 36, 42, 48, 147–149; under nutritional treatment plan, 176
Weiss, Dr. Norman, 15

Xanax®, 65, 68–69, 101–102, 103, 105, 208, 210
xanthines, 94

yeast infection, 47, 224–225; self-diagnosis test for, 225; treatment of, 225
Yen, Dr. S. S., 221
yoga, 62

Zoloft®, 212